Impact of Divorce on the Extended Family

Impact of Divorce on the Extended Family

Esther Oshiver Fisher, Editor

Journal of Divorce
Volume 5, Numbers 1/2

The Haworth Press
New York

The Haworth Press, Inc., 28 East 22 Street, New York, NY 10010.

Library of Congress Cataloging in Publication Data

Main entry under title:

Impact of divorce on the extended family.

    (Journal of divorce; v. 5, no. 1/2)
    Includes bibliographical references.
    1. Divorce–Addresses, essays, lectures. 2. Family–Addresses, essays, lectures.
I. Fisher, Esther Oshiver. II. Series
K10.08595   v. 5, no. 1/2   306.8'9'05s   81-20207
[HQ84]   [306.8'9]   AACR2
ISBN 0-917724-43-7

EDITOR

ESTHER OSHIVER FISHER, JD, EdD, *Marriage and Divorce Counselor, New York, NY*

EDITOR-ELECT

CRAIG A. EVERETT, PhD, *Tucson, Arizona*

EDITORIAL BOARD

Impact of Divorce
on the
Extended Family

Journal of Divorce
Volume 5, Numbers 1/2

CLINICAL PRACTICE

Impact of Divorce on the Extended Family

PREFACE

The economic and sociological development of the nuclear family—husband, wife and their children—as against the earlier home-industrial extended family has brought to the nuclear family a plethora of research, theory development, and clinical attention. Professional concern for today's extended family has lagged.

By concept and definition, the nuclear family makes for a relatively closed circuit of relationships—husband, wife and children. The circuit, thus structured, postulates a crescendo of internal expectations, demands and disappointments followed by frustrations, angers and resentments that frequently lead to divorce. The result has been that the nuclear family has received our primary and almost exclusive professional study and concern, particularly in regard to divorce.

We speak about divorce as having reached epidemic proportions but have largely ignored that an epidemic is not confined to those who are initially distressed.

When I contemplated the quantum of professional writing with respect to the marital couple and their children in relation to the onset and impact of divorce and the apparent paucity of study as to what was concomitantly happening to other family members, I chose to initiate the present special study of the impact of divorce upon other immediate family members that make up the extended family related to the divorcing or divorced couple, to wit, their parents, siblings and in-laws, and those other relatives with whom the couple has had a close, on-going relationship.

As editor of the *Journal of Divorce*, I express my appreciation to the scholars and professionals who accepted my invitation to participate and the challenge it presented in this relatively uncharted area. I particularly thank Craig Everett, PhD, and Wilbert Sykes, MD, for their editorial reviews and constructive suggestions.

In accord with the overall purpose of the *Journal of Divorce*, the studies here presented are from various disciplines.

Of course, it is my hope that this work may become the harbinger of further professional attention and research as to the impact of divorce in the nuclear family upon the extended family.

Esther Oshiver Fisher, JD, EdD
Editor

DIVORCE AND THE DYNAMICS
OF THE FAMILY KINSHIP SYSTEM

Michael Duffy

ABSTRACT. Little research exists on the dynamics of relationships within the extended family after divorce and remarriage. Several related methodological/conceptual issues are presented in explanation of this gap in research: the persistence of a nuclear mythology surrounding the family, differences in the focus of sociological and psychological research, and the neglect of research on qualitative aspects of family interactions. On the basis of the existing limited research and clinical data, an account is given of general and specific dynamic patterns within post-divorce and post-remarriage interactions in the extended family.

This article examines the dynamic patterns in relationships between members of the extended family after divorce and after subsequent remarriage. While there has been a modest amount of research on the effects of divorce on spouses and children (the "nuclear" family), very little attention has been given to the effects of divorce upon the extended family. More pertinently, almost no research data exists in the area of psychological dynamics of post-divorce relationships in the extended family. This is critical since it leaves clinicians without reliable data or models in their work with divorced families.

It is by no means accidental that this situation exists. Thus, prior to

Michael Duffy, PhD, is affiliated with the Department of Educational Psychology, College of Education, Texas A & M University, College Station, Texas 77843. The author wishes to thank Mr. Douglas Moller for his suggestions and editorial assistance.

3

examining what is known of post-divorce and post-re-marriage family dynamics, this article will first outline some of the reasons for these omissions in research. There are several related methodological issues which have dogged the progress of research in this area.

The Composition of the Extended Family System

The Nuclear/Extended Family Debate

At the forefront of the problem is the question of whether the extended kin network actually exists in American society—at least in any functionally meaningful sense? This is clearly an issue of fundamental importance; if, as some have suggested, the extended family is little more than a vestige of pre-industrial society, then divorce can be expected to have minimal impact on the larger family network. If the extended family is indeed alive and well, then it will not only be significantly affected by marital disruption, but will provide an important resource to distressed members.

There is little doubt that the American family has undergone considerable change during this century and that it differs sharply from families in other cultural traditions (Mead, 1971; Uzoka, 1979). The nuclear family unit, consisting of the two spouses and their dependent children, is certainly the focal point of any larger family system.* Relationships between members have evolved in a voluntary rather than an obligatory form (Johnson, 1977). The proportion of older generations living under the same roof as younger family members has dwindled to approximately 4% and 14% of older men and women respectively (Mindel, 1979). Perhaps underlying all of these characteristics is the financial independence of family members. It remains to be seen if the trend dispersion and economic independence will be affected by a recessionary economy.

In the 1940's these changing trends were characterized by the notion of the "isolated nuclear family" (Parsons, 1949). Not only was the increasing autonomy of the nuclear family recognized, but it was considered to be "functionally atomistic" and isolated from the wider kinfolk network (Zimmerman, 1947). This analysis, largely the work of cultural anthropologists and sociologists has had a profound influence on both scientific and popular conceptions of the contemporary family.

---

*There is some evidence, however, that the dominant and central family unit has always been the nuclear family. While the multigenerational household may have been normatively accepted, life expectancy rates made it uncommon (Mindel, 1979).

While it has largely been proved inadequate (if not inaccurate) by later research (Shanas, 1965), it remains a pervasive influence in the area of clinical practice. Thus, there has been a generalized dearth of research into transgenerational dynamics within extended kin networks. When divorce occurs within the nuclear family unit, clinicians rarely focus on its effects upon the extended family.

While the conception of the isolated nuclear family derived largely from an over-reliance on quantitative accounts of intergenerational contacts, this quantitative data itself has been shown to be misleading. Shanas (1979), in analyzing nationwide probability surveys of elderly over 1957, 1962 and 1975, was able to put to rest the myth of alienation in the extended family. Four of every five non-institutionalized persons over 65 have living children and most have regular and even daily contact with children and relatives. While older people may no longer live in the same household with a child (mostly by choice), they often live in the same neighborhood or city with at least one relative, and over 80% have at least weekly contact. The family remains the main support system for the older person; and this help is reciprocated in almost equal proportion. This situation remains even with the advent of external supports such as Social Security, Medicaid, and Medicare. Thus, even in simple quantitative terms of "physical" intergenerational contact, the notion of an isolated nuclear family is not supported by the facts.

Quantitative versus Qualitative

That the qualitative dimension of extended family relationships has been almost totally neglected is perhaps the major element in the growth and persistence of nuclear mythology. Even recent conceptual revisions such as "the modified extended family" (Litwak, 1965) are based heavily on the *incidence* of contacts between family members. Few researchers have addressed the *qualitative* aspects of those relationships. Although it is fairly obvious that frequency of contact is not simply correlated with the quality of that contact, studies have been "essentially devoid of investigations of feeling or affect" (Wilen, 1979). Measures of contact alone do not illustrate the motivational dynamics of that contact, nor its intensity or importance (Spicer, 1975).

While there are numerous statistical and demographic studies of divorce, there are few which examine dynamic aspects of interpersonal adjustment to divorce (Dawson, 1979). A notable and welcome exception to this is the work of Wallerstein and Kelly (1974, 1975, 1976).

Their work, however, is focused largely on the psychological effects of divorce on spouses and children within the nuclear family unit.

A couple of examples of typical methodologies will illustrate this utilization of incidence of contact as a measure of intergenerational relationships in divorced families. In a study of kinship interaction after divorce, Spicer's (1975) key measure of contact was home visiting, indicated by responses to the question, "How often do you and your parents visit each other in your homes?" (p. 114). Similarly, Anspach (1976), asked study participants, "How many times in the past seven days did you have contact with (relative)?". On the basis of quantitatively decreasing indications of this type of contact, both authors perceived a weakening of kinship interaction, at least with former spouse's kindred. Jacobson (1978) studied the relation between "time-lost" with absent fathers and children's adjustment to divorce. There is no doubt that such measures of incidence and length of contact are of great value; it is, however, misleading to assume that the greater the physical interaction, the closer or more meaningful are the relationships. Also, this approach may neglect to take into account greater geographic dispersion and more flexible patterns of interaction. Children, for example, may visit the absent father's kin less frequently but for longer periods (Furstenberg, 1979). This cannot be taken to imply that relationships are qualitatively weaker.

Clearly, incidence and length of contact are associated with quality and meaningfulness of relationships. But it is not a parallel correlation. Quantity of contact is rather a *mediator* of quality. Relationships will rarely be good unless a minimum of physical contact is assured. It should be noted, however, that "physical" contact today can be achieved in a number of ways, not the least of which is the telephone.

In an attempt to preserve the qualitative as well as quantitative dimension of interaction, Furstenberg (1979) utilized an unstructured question format. This allowed study participants to elaborate on the quality and meaning of interaction with extended kin.

Sociological View versus Psychological View

It will probably not have escaped the reader's attention that in describing these discrepant (but potentially complementary) approaches, we have also described customary differences in the focus and methods of sociology and psychology. Credit for development of theory and research in extended family networks must be given to family sociologists. Neglect of the "psychological-affective-transactional" aspects of those networks (Uzoka, 1979) probably results from lack of attention by psychologists. Where there is much overlap between the two disciplines, it is probably fair to make the following distinction in analysis of the extended family: sociology has largely provided an "outside-structural" view of intergenerational relations; it is the task of psychology to provide the complementary "inside-dynamic" view. While psychologists, and mainly clinicians, have contributed significantly to a dynamic systems view of nuclear family disruptions, they have tended to neglect the reactions of members of the extended family system to those members of disruptions, particularly those that end in divorce.

Enter the Clinician

In one sense, the distinction being drawn is not between disciplines as such, but rather between methodological orientation. Thus it is the clinical practice perspective (involving not all psychologists, nor exclusive of sociologists) which is reasonably likely to generate testable hypotheses relating to the dynamics of the extended family system. Herein lies the problem: few clinicians systematically conduct research, and few researchers have a clinical perspective—even broadly defined. The result: untested clinical insight is rightly held suspect, and the research hypotheses and data of academic researchers are often unsuccessful in conveying the richness and complexity of individual and family psychodynamics. Cooperation and integration of specialties is critical in the development of reliable and relevant data on family interaction, or in any other area of enquiry. Without this integration of effort, academic researchers produce "collectivistic" data which is marginally useful in clinical practice (O'Brien, 1977) and clinicians run the risk of overgeneralizing from clinical data. Scientific enquiry will best emanate from questions arising in actual human relations (typically in "clinical" situations), thus avoiding the neglect of idiosyncrasy and individual differences. Too much *a priori* suspicion of clinical insight has inhibited research into its validity or generalizability. It is arguable that clinical dynamics, or even psychopathologies, are extensions or extreme portrayals of normal dynamics (Maudsley, 1977) and cannot be neglected in the analysis of interpersonal transactions.

What follows is a composite picture of psychological aspects of extended family relationships following divorce and subsequent remarriage. It is the "inside-dynamic" perspective on these issues. It is a picture gleaned from very limited existing data and from personal clinical experience. At best it represents a limited "state of the art."

Patterns of Continuity and Change in the Family Kinship System

Post Divorce

Spicer (1975) and Anspach (1976), on the basis of quantitative measure of contact, have noted a weakening of kin relationships following divorce. Affection and interaction between each divorcee and their own parents (consanguines) continues after divorce, but the relations with their parents- and relatives-in-law (affines) is weakened. Social relations of children with paternal kin (grandparents, uncles, aunts) are mediated through their degree of contact with the absent father, which has typically been very limited.

Reflecting on the incidence and effects of divorce in the United States, Mead (1971) commented:

> We have constructed a family system which depends on fidelity, lifelong monogamy and the survival of both parents. But we have never made adequate social provision for the security and identity of the children if that marriage is broken, as it so often was in the past by death or desertion, and as it so often is in the present by death or divorce. We have, in fact, ... saddled ourselves with a system that won't work (p. 115).

This is in sharp distinction to the family system of other societies,

> Where children learn to turn to one relative for solace, and to another for the mastery of a skill, the continuum of the marriage of their own parents is not so essential. Identity, security, adult backing in youth, and youthful help in old age are all assured by wider family ties (p. 114).

There is no doubt that divorce had and still has a deleterious effect on the family; the evidence for this continues to be overwhelming—even to the extent that divorce, as a cure, can often be "worse than the disease" (Welch and Granvold, 1977). However, these analyses, while rightly pointing to the stress engendered by marital disruption, perhaps fail to recognize the flexibility and gradual adaptation that is inherent in the dynamic family system. Cross-cultural studies have demonstrated that kinship structures confronted with advanced industrialization and technology do not dissolve, but evolve and adjust (Quinn, 1979). The same process may well be present in the kin network following divorce. What can be viewed as structural decline and dissolution of the extended family network, can from another perspective be regarded as the conflictual struggle to find new forms of interrelationships. It is perhaps significant that the perspectives of Spicer, Anspach and Mead represent the earlier part of this decade. It is at least plausible that in the last decade and in years to come, the disruptive effect of divorce on the extended family may be lessened. Mead (1971), with the insight of a great anthropologist, urged the development of two kinds of marriage relationships: (1) without children—without the obligatory quality of emotional and economic interdependence; (2) with children—where, through the child, parents have an irreversible, indissoluble relationship with each other, regardless of the state of the marriage contract. In this situation the well-being of children and supportive kin relationships would be better preserved. Again, it is not unreasonable to perceive the prophetic quality of this notion in the current development of more flexible custody arrangements which allow continuing parental interaction in the rearing of children.

Furstenberg (1979) in an excellent case study on the restructuring of kinship ties, points out that earlier studies examined only the effects of divorce on the relationships between adults and former affines. This, of course, fails to recognize that kin members may relate independently to children regardless of the state of the divorcees' relationship. These are consanguineous relationships, and, for example, grandparents often make strenuous efforts to maintain close ties with their grandchildren in the face of parental conflict. And through the grandparents the children often maintain regular contact with uncles, aunts and cousins. The grandparent-grandchild relationship thus has a key mediating role in the continuance of kin networks that has often been neglected in research suggesting the demise of extended kin networks.

This may also be true of other dyadic relationships after divorce. "I might, for example, consider my ex-sister-in-law a member of my family either because she *was* my brother's wife, because she *is* my nephew's mother, or merely because I feel close to her" (Furstenberg, (1979) p. 19). Such relationships, while perhaps infrequent and unidentified by studies stressing degree rather than importance of contact, may well presage future adaptations.

If we can assume that, for a significant proportion of persons, adult personal attachment and emotional investment are primarily accomplished in marriage (Welch and Granvold, 1977), then divorce is clearly very disruptive at a personal level. More pertinent to this argument, the inevitable preoccupation with personal hurt and needs will seriously limit the divorcees' ability to give supportive care to their children or older parents (Weed, 1979). Predictably, the personal adjustment of children generally declines in the first year following divorce, and then, at least for girls, shows a steady improvement in the second year (Heatherington, 1978). But it has been shown in general (Shanas, 1979) that older people are not simply the *receivers* of help in the extended family. They *give* almost as much assistance as they receive, and what they contribute is not just "the wisdom of the ages," but significant and practical assistance such as child-care, housework and cooking, as well as important economic and personal support. Older parents, uncles, aunts and grandparents frequently provide material and emotional support, relieve some of the stress of child care, and often provide a "neutral zone" where the divorcees can more calmly exercise their parental role (Furstenberg, 1979).

The importance of older generations in the extended family will probably increase as four- and even five-generation families become common. One of the emerging problems of this expanding network is that middle-aged parents may face emotional (and financial) responsibility for as many as two older and two younger generations. For these persons, divorcing adult children (or parents) represent a special challenge to their willingness to remain involved in the family network.

The stress of mutual caretaking within these larger family systems is partly offset by the availability of social services. While frequently blamed for the erosion of ties between extended kin, social services in fact often alleviate material burdens, allowing family members to invest more energy in emotional support (Johnson, 1977; Quinn, 1979).

Post-Remarriage

If the period following divorce can be seen to offer an opportunity for kinship ties to assert themselves in new ways and to reassert themselves in a stronger, deeper way, the period following remarriage of a divorced spouse presents even more striking changes (both quantitative and qualitative) in the kinship system. Moreover, while the post-divorce period allows for important reforms within a family unit which has undergone stress and disorder, remarriage can signal a genuine revolution in the family system wherein not only are roles redefined but new roles are discovered and invented.

Family kinship interactions are at least potentially increased when one or both divorcees remarry. Examined from the child's point of view, for example, the new family network has expanded enormously. The child, through parent remarriages, can acquire new sets of grandparents and a host of new brothers and sisters, uncles, aunts and cousins, not to mention a range of more distant but possibly significant relatives. And even if the child has no blood ties to the new "step" family, culturally they are permitted to, and frequently do, think of these relations as equivalent to blood relatives (Furstenberg, 1979).

It is true that sometimes step-relatives are seen as a replacement of the original family, but they can also be rightly viewed as an addition to the family system (Bohannon, 1971)—thus providing a range of new resources. Indeed, Furstenberg (1979) has made the fascinating observation that "remarriage recreates a kinship configuration which disappeared several generations ago" (p. 31). Further, it is not unreasonable to suggest that the extensive post-remarriage network bears resemblance to family constellations where polygamy is the cultural norm. In this latter case children (and spouses) are likely to view the extensive kin network as a relational resource rather than a source of bitter competition.

Herein lies an important issue. However regrettable it may be considered, divorce and remarriage are facts of contemporary life—and possibly represent a fairly stable trend. It seems critical that reconstituted family networks be "normalized" as an institutional form such that this societal "recognition" will encourage family growth rather than conflict. The legal process, while it mandates continued parental involvement through the mechanism of economic child support, provides only minimally for emotional obligation of absent parents. It might be suggested that contact between ex-spouses (and their families) should not only be "permitted" through visitation rights, but encouraged. This institutional recognition of the indissoluability of the parental role might have welcome consequences; the new spouse, for instance, may feel less threatened and competitive in the continued involvement with the "old" family since such involvement would be considered "normal."

Mead (1971), observing the negative historical connotations of "step" terminology, urged the development of a new language. In support of this possibility she points to the facility of children in developing affectionate but different names for their various grandparents. The awkwardness of available terminology ("my stepsibling's grandparents") certainly underlines the need for normalcy in the large kin-networks created by remarriage.

There are some signs of the evolution of new forms of relationships in the post-remarriage network. The very lack of norms for appropriate and permissible ways to relate has allowed a greater flexibility to develop (Johnson, 1977; Furstenberg, 1979). Obligations are unspecific so that maintenance of a relationship is not tied to frequency of contact. The particular form of a relationship can thus respond to idiosyncratic preferences. As Satir (1972) has pointed out, the fact that family members do not live under the same roof does not imply that they do not contribute to each others growth. And this physical autonomy may, in fact, contribute to warm and less obligatory relationships.

With decreasing birth rates, remarriage has an interesting side effect; it potentially "distributes a decreasing pool of children among a larger circle of adults" (Furstenberg, 1979 p. 31). This relationship with the children in turn can have the effect of strengthening the relationships of adults who would otherwise have no reason for contact. This, serendipitously, helps counteract an unfortunate tendency sometimes reinforced by clinicians: the belief that the strengthening of the new family must necessarily involve breaking ties with the old family (Kleinman, 1979). Spouses often fail to recognize that their need to "separate" from one another is different from their child's need to continue both parental and familial relationships. In this way children are often victims of adults' perceptions of what is inevitable in the divorce process. In fact, it is probably true that children's needs are best-served the more extensive is the kinship system. If not influenced by parents' negative attitudes, the child can find support in the wide array of new relationships provided by remarriage.

Specific Dynamics

Post-Divorce

Many psychological interactions can be regarded as expressions of a dynamic realignment of roles and power within the post-divorce family network.

Within the dynamics of the family network a prevalent theme is the importance of implicitly assigned *roles*, and especially the reallocation or reversal of roles. As children become adult there is a normative, developmental rebalancing of dependency roles with parents. In one sense, a criterion of maturity is the ability to perceive a parent as an equal or even as a dependent. Divorce often interrupts this process, in that young adults may become again increasingly dependent on parents and sometimes on their own children. Thus a daughter may rely heavily on her mother for support and decisions regarding her divorce. Another variation on this theme is the development of a counter-dependence to cope with the growing threat to autonomy engendered by emotional and economic reliance on parents (Welch and Granvold, 1977). In turn, children of divorce often develop a pseudo-maturity as they try sympathetically to provide for their parents' needs. In clinical practice this author has often noted the isolation and anger of early adolescent children as they try to cope with the "neo-adolescent" dating and sexual explorations of divorced parents.

The dynamics of *role-reversal* can be seen in the exercise of parental discipline following divorce. The absent father frequently surrenders the disciplinarian role to the mother who may subsequently find that this unwelcome role thrusts her into a struggle with her children—making her a prime target for their displaced anger at their father. The absent father, meanwhile, removed from the stresses of marital conflict, may develop a richer, affectional relationship with his children (Wallerstein and Kelly, 1975). This is reminiscent of the tranquil characteristics of child-grandparent relationships where minimal responsibility permits greater mutual enjoyment.

In general the female role is important in the maintenance of the family kinship system. Women typically place more value on kin relationships than do men, who emphasize friendships with peers (Ward, 1979). For this reason it has been noted that, for men, bereavement, without the benefit of developed kin relationships, can be acutely lonely. Wilen (1979) has depicted the woman as the "primary kinkeeper" to indicate her role in preserving and strengthening the kinship network. This emphasizes again the importance of the grandmother in marital disruption.

For the child, divorce can seriously interrupt the development of *phase-specific roles and relationships*. Wallerstein and Kelly (1976) stress that "divorce necessarily affects the freedom of the child to keep major attention riveted outside the family" (p. 257). This often has the effect of decreasing the number and quality of outside relationships and distracting attention from academic achievement. Particularly important during adolescence is the tendency of divorce to interrupt the process of "decathecting" emotional ties to parents. In this situation the adolescent may retreat into inappropriate emotional dependency or rush into pseudo-autonomy and premature sexual experiences. Younger children in the latency period typically strive to preserve a poise in the face of painful feelings. And while there is no consistent evidence that children feel responsible for their parents' divorce, they often experience anger, fear of rejection, loyalty conflicts and a shaken sense of identity (Wallerstein and Kelly, 1976). This situation strongly suggests the need for maintaining consistent parental involvement despite divorce and the value of a strong kin network.

The *role of parents-in-law* in the dynamics of divorce has also been seriously underestimated—mostly because of an assumption that emotional ties between spouse and in-laws are minimal. In fact, because of deficiencies in their own parental relationships, many persons adopt affines as "new parents." In a series of clinical case studies, Lager (1977) illustrates the potential importance of relations with parents-in-law. He points out that researchers and therapists rarely consider the relationship significant and often miss the fact that in-laws are an important support system. Further, they are occasionally critically involved in the process of marital disruption itself. On the one hand, for example, spouses may be able to rework personal issues with their parent-in-law which they had not resolved with their own parent. On the other hand, termination or deterioration of the parent-in-law relationship may directly contribute to marital disruption. Lager cites the case of a divorce which followed shortly after the death of a significant mother-in-law to whom the divorcee had effectively been "married." In a real sense, parents-in-law can be a "second chance family" (p. 19), variously important in the precipitation and resolution of family disruption. This is clearly at variance with the image of in-law relations being of simple "nuisance" value as a thorn in the side of marital relations.

The *distribution and exercise of power* after divorce remains, as always, the most pervasive of family dynamics—possibly at the base of all other dynamics. From a dynamic and legal standpoint, the "adversary" system is symptomatic of an inherent struggle for power during divorce. Thus, problematic issues are contested rather than negotiated, as would be encouraged by mediation approaches. The interruption of established roles and "rules" necessarily generates a struggle for redistribution of personal power in the extended family. Issues, like the well-being of children, rather than being resolved on the merits of the case, become vehicles for the establishment of power. There is an important issue here. While a mediation approach, encouraging the negotiation of issues, must eventually predominate if the power distribution is to be rebalanced, there may well be a need for a conflictual stage that must be experienced. In this sense there may be an implicit wisdom in the adversarial stance of the more traditional legal system. How often have couples "intelligently discussed" their divorce and custody arrangements, only to end up in the courts at a later time requesting a settlement decision?

Newsome (1977) found that much of the "bargaining" in the post-divorce situation fits well within the framework of *exchange theory*. In terms of the parents' continuing involvement in the family system he found that: (1) the greater the inputs of the divorced father, the greater his outcomes over children from whom he has been separated; (2) the greater the inputs of the divorced father, the more positive the sentiments of the ex-wife; (3) the more positive the sentiments of the ex-wife, the greater the outcomes of the divorced father. Thus, while anger and conflict will initially be present, mutually satisfying solutions to the sharing of power and responsibility can be reached through "quid pro quo" negotiations. Johnson (1977) similarly found evidence of the operation of exchange theory in the kinship system of Japanese-Americans through the operation of indebtedness and reciprocity among members. Such exchanges, especially in divorce, serve the purpose of "empowering" family members once again and thus contributing to conflict resolution.

Post-Remarriage

While the dynamics discussed above remain pertinent, remarriage raises several special issues.

One of the complicating factors in the development of the new family system is the *expectations* that derive from the families of origin and from the painful experience of divorce (Whiteside and Auerbach, 1978). Because of the mistakes and unreconciled conflicts of the past, the new spouses feel that, "this time it has to work." Even less realistically, spouses sometimes are hopeful that this second marriage will approach the state of Nirvana (Satir, 1972). Both naive optimism and excessive pessimism work against the chances of success. Realism, rather, dictates a clear recognition of the problems to be faced. Often both spouses and their children have been through a long period of stress and may not have fully grasped, or changed, the circumstances that led to their divorce. A period of gradual accommodation is required during which expectations are kept in low profile.

Armed with grandiose expectations, a step-parent often feels required immediately to love and be loved by the step-child. As an interloper, this is rarely possible, and the step-parent will only become integrated into the family if he or she can understand, and tolerate, the need to build relationships gradually. Associated with the expectations of immediately loving and being loved by a step-child is the pressure on the step-parent to substitute for the biological parent. This is neither possible nor desirable. While it is necessary to assume some parental characteristics, such as control and discipline, for most the role of the step-parent will at best supplement, not replace the role of the original parent.

When new spouses are less hopeful of success in their reconstituted family they may approach the marital bond with an extreme caution that inhibits the development of family relationships. (Particularly, it should be said that to approach remarriage with a naive optimism may itself be a covert defense against fear of failure). Pritchard (1977) found that this caution led spouses to relate with an indirect, non-confrontative style and with unwillingness to exchange explicit information on matters of importance.

This reticence in risking intimacy with the new spouse may lead the mother, for example, to redevelop an intense interdependence with her own children (Messinger, 1976), thus producing closed systems within the family. Kleinman (1979) points out that the reconstituted family will frequently divide into the original sub-units when faced with initial distrust or later tension. From a clinical point of view the hardening of these divisions within the family represent one of the most difficult obstacles to change.

In such circumstances, the children may feel increased resentment, not only at the step-parent, but also at the parent— who may be judged responsible for the divorce and ensuing alienation (Kleinman, 1979). This resentment may be exacerbated by the child's inability to share or even comprehend the parent's sense of joy and relief in the new relationship. Feeling powerless and alienated, such children may attempt to exert some form of control over the situation by challenging the quality of parenting. "Watch how you treat me or I'll go and live with my father," is a familiar example of this dynamic (Whiteside, 1978).

For adolescents, there may be new sources of sexual tension in the reconstituted family. Mead (1971) has pointed out that familiarity and intimacy between step-relations are not counterbalanced by protective, deeply felt taboos regarding sexual behavior. The reconstituted family is a recent enough phenomenon that social norms simply have not yet developed. Sexual tension may exist between step-parent and adolescent child and between step-siblings (often thinly disguised as aggression).

Conclusion

The events of divorce and remarriage clearly have a significant effect on the dynamics of relationship and adaptive capacity of the extended family. Such events generate the need for a series of special transitions which challenge sensitivity and flexibility, but may lead to new and enriched relationships.

As the incidence of divorce increases, there emerges a critical need for data which accurately reflects both quantitative and qualitative aspects of family interactions. This in turn challenges clinicians and researchers to develop a mutual understanding of critical variables if the qualitative changes in contemporary family life are to be adequately investigated.

REFERENCES

Anspach, D.F. Kinship and divorce. *Journal of Marriage and the Family*, 1976, *38*, 323-330.

Bohannon, P. Divorce chains, households of remarriage, and multiple divorcers. In, P. Bohannon (Ed.), *Divorce and After: An Analysis of the Emotional and Social Problems of Divorcees*. New York: Anchor Books, 1971.

Dawson, D.R. Selected factors in divorce and separation adjustment. *Diss. Abst. Int.*, 1979, *39* (7-A), 4056.

Furstenberg, F.F., Jr. Remarriage and intergenerational relations. Paper presented at a workshop on Stability and Change, Annapolis, Maryland, March, 1979.

Heatherington, E.M. Family interaction and the social, emotional and cognitive development of children following divorce. *Resources in Education*, 1978, ED156328.

Jacobson, D.S. The impact of marital separation/divorce on children: I. Parent-child separation and child adjustment. *Journal of Divorce*, 1978, vol. l(4).

Johnson, C.L. Interdependence reciprocity and indebtedness: An analysis of Japanese American kinship relations. *Journal of Marriage and the Family*, 1977, *39*, 351-363.

Kelly, J.B. & Wallerstein, J.S. The effects of parental divorce: Experiences of the child in early latency. *American Journal of Orthopsychiatry*, 1976, *46*, 20-32.

Kleinman, J., Rosenberg, E. & Whiteside, M. Common developmental tasks in forming reconstituted families. *Journal of Marital and Family Therapy*, 1979, *5*, 79-86.

Lager, E. Parents-in-law: Failure and divorce in a second chance family. *Journal of Marriage and Family Counseling*, 1977, *3*, 19-23.

Litwak, E. Extended kin relations in an industrial democratic society. In E. Shanas and G.F. Streib (Eds.), *Social Structure and the family: gerontological relations*. Englewood Cliffs, N.J.: Prentice-Hall, 1965.

Maudsley, H. Physiology and pathology of the mind (N.Y. 1867), available in *Significant Contributions to the History of Psychology* (Series C. Vol. IV). D.N. Robinson (Ed.), Washington, D.C.: University Publications of America, 1977.

Mead, M. Anomalies in American post-divorce relationships. In P. Bohannon (Ed.), *Divorce and After: An Analysis of Emotional Social Problems of Divorcees.* New York: Anchor Books, 1971.

Messinger, L. Remarriage between divorced people with children from previous marriages: A proposal for preparation for remarriage. *Journal of Marriage and Family Counseling*, 1976, *2*, 193-200.

Mindel, C.H. Multigenerational family households: Recent trends and implications for the future. *The Gerontologist*, 1979, *19*, 456-463.

Newsome, O.D. Post-divorce interaction: An explanation using exchange theory. *Diss. Abst. Int.*, 1977, *37* (12-A, Pt. 1), 8001.

O'Brien, D.J. & Garland, T.N. Bridging the gap between theory, research, practice and policy making: The case of interaction with kin after divorce. *Resources in Education* (RIE), 1977, ED153101.

Parsons, T. The Social Structure of the Family. In R.N. Anshen (Ed.), *The Family: Its functions and destiny.* New York: Harper, 1949.

Pritchard, J.W. Divorce-remarriage: An investigation of the effects of divorce and related variables on the communication style of reconstituted families. *Diss. Abst. Int.*, 1977, *38* (1-B), 375.

Quinn, W.H. & Hughston, G.A. The family as a natural support system for the aged. Paper presented at the Annual Meeting of the Gerontological Society, Washington, D.C., November, 1979.

Satir, V. *Peoplemaking.* Palo Alto: Science and Behavior Books, Inc., 1972.

Shanas, E. and G.F. Streib (Eds.), Social structure and the family: gerontological relations. Englewood Cliffs, N.J.: Prentice-Hall, 1965.

Shanas, E. Social myth as hypothesis: The case of the family relations of old people. *The Gerontologist*, Vol. 19, No. l, 1979.

Spicer, J.W. & Hampe, G.D. Kinship interaction after divorce. *Journal of Marriage and the Family*, 1975, *37*, 113-119.

Uzoka, A.F. The myth of the nuclear family: Historical background and clinical implications. *American Psychologist*, 1979, *34*, 1095-1106.

Wallerstein, J.S. & Kelly, J.B. The effects of parental divorce: The adolescent experience. In J. Anthony & C. Koupernik (Eds.), *The Child in His Family: Children at Psychiatric Risk.* New York: John Wiley & Sons, 1974.

Wallerstein, J.S. & Kelly, J.B. The effects of parental divorce: Experiences of the preschool child. *Journal of the American Academy of Child Psychiatry*, 1975, *14*, 601-616.

Wallerstein, J.S. & Kelly, J.B. The effects of parental divorce: Experiences in later latency. *American Journal of Orthopsychiatry*, 1976, *46*, 256-269.

Ward, R.A. *The Aging Experience: An Introduction to Social Gerontology.* New York: J.B. Lippincott Company, 1979.

Weed, J.A. Implications of divorce and remarriage for the physical health of the aged and their adult children. Paper presented at the Annual Meeting of the Gerontological Society, Washington, D.C., November, 1979.

Welch, G.J. & Granvold, D.K. Seminars for separated/divorced: An educational approach to post-divorce adjustment. *Journal of Sex & Marital Therapy*, 1977, Vol. 3, No. 1, 31-39.

Whiteside, M.F. & Auerbach, L.S. Can the daughter of my father's new wife be my sister? *Journal of Divorce*, Vol. 1(3), 1978, 271-283.

Wilen, J.B. Changing relationships among grandparents, parents, and their young children. Paper presented at the Annual Meeting of the Gerontological Society, Washington, D.C., November, 1979.

Zimmerman, C.C. *Family and Civilization.* New York: Harper and Row, 1947.

DIVORCE, THE FAMILY LIFE CYCLE, AND ITS EMPIRICAL DEFICIENCIES

William Bytheway

ABSTRACT. This paper presents some descriptive data which places divorce in the general content of family histories. It examines the occurrence of divorce: (1) within complete marital careers; (2) within a section of the extended family, including siblings and cousins, as well as parents, uncles and aunts; and (3) within the children of older persons. The data is drawn from a unique source that records complete family histories within the British peerage. The analysis demonstrates wide variations in the experience of divorce within the family — particularly among older persons. It also shows that the majority of individuals in this population did have some personal experience. It argues that divorce has to be considered in the context of general life-long processes, and to this end the family life cycle proves to be an unhelpful and invalid conceptual device.

Many studies in family sociology have taken the nuclear family as a starting point along with the corresponding dynamic, the family life cycle. The concept of the extended family has come to be identified in this context with the four parents of the married couple of the nuclear family: the grandparents. Insofar as the family life cycle eventually leaves the two parents as sole remaining members, their children all

William Bytheway, PhD received his doctorate in Sociology in 1973 from the University of Keele, has written numerous articles on Health and Old Age, and is on the Editorial Board of Sociology of Health and Illness. He has been Senior Research Fellow since 1975 at the Medical Sociology Research Centre, University College of Swansea, Wales, United Kingdom.

having left to marry, it naturally follows that some relationship must continue between them and the newly established nuclear families of their children. The concept of the extended family neatly allows for this continuing relationship: the basic concept of the family can be "extended" to add to the nuclear family the denuded families from which the two adult members come. This conceptualization reaffirms the philosophy that older persons should and do remain as integrated members of the wider society, based as it is upon the concept of "family."

While this model represents an ideal which one would not necessarily wish to refute, it is based upon a range of assumptions each of which is of doubtful empirical validity. These assumptions (which admittedly are only loosely formulated and rarely applied in a rigorous way) are: (i) that a marriage does produce children, (ii) that children do leave the nuclear family through marriage, (iii) that a marriage does survive unbroken into a shared old age, and (iv) that the aged husband dies first, the wife surviving a few more years as an unremarrying widow. It is still true that in most Western societies most marriages do produce children, that most children do marry in early adulthood and that most marriages do remain intact for a long period of time, and that most are eventually broken by the death of the husband. It is doubtful, however, whether or not most nuclear families succeed in fulfilling this ideal in all these different ways. In Bytheway (1979), I showed that in respect to one particular contemporary population this was not the case. The ideal sequence of there being more than one child in the family, all marrying before the death of the husband/father which in turn preceded the death of the unremarried widow/mother characterized only 6 percent of 934 families.

Divorce does not occur in the ideal family life cycle—marriages are assumed to remain intact until broken by death in old age. Moreover the study of divorce has tended to be seen as separate from the study of the family. Nevertheless when the subject of divorce is discussed in the context of the family, there is a widespread belief, supported by the association of divorce with age that is apparent in available statistics, that divorce is associated with the processes of adjustment to early married life. Given two married generations within a family, it is the younger generation which will tend to be associated with the possibility of divorce.

In the context of the extended family outlined above, interest will center upon the interrelationships between the divorcing couple of the nuclear family and their parents, rather than upon a divorcing couple and their married children. In particular, attention will be focused upon the possible interplay between child divorce and parental adjustments to the "problems" of old age, such as bereavement.

This inter-play can be predicted on the basis of demographic data showing the statistical associations that age has with marriage, child-bearing, divorce and death (Bytheway 1977b). It is further anticipated by case material arising from varied sources. To take just one example, the British poet and novelist A. Alvarez, who has written a popular book on the subject of suicide, was reported in the Sunday Times of 30.3.80 to be working on a book on divorce. The report reads: "His research has taken him all round Europe . . . 'So many people seem to model their married life on a fantasy of their parents' marriage. You'd be surprised how many women suddenly decide on a divorce when their fathers die.' " Without more information it is impossible to assess the validity of this claim, but the important point is that the Sunday Times' journalist described this observation as "fascinating." The fact is that neither the overly-simple demographic statistics, nor the knowledge gained through case work is sufficient to provide an empirical description of how divorce and other events in the histories of extended families are statistically interrelated.

The purpose of this paper is simply to present such empirical material. It seemed appropriate to focus attention upon the many varied sequences of events in the extended family in which divorce occurs, rather than upon the calculation of age-specific rates or indeed upon the testing of exotic hypotheses such as that put forward by Alvarez. The data is drawn from the same population of 934 families used in Bytheway (1979).

There are two aspects of this population which must be fully appreciated. The first is that the population was intended to possess the following characteristic: each family is "recently completed" in the sense that both the parents of the defining nuclear family have died, the last dying between 1955 and 1970. In other words, a family is defined by a married couple and the children (if any) of the marriage, and it is described as completed when the surviving member of the marriage dies.

This was the intended population. Unfortunately, the source of data (to be described below) was such that when the married couple had divorced it was frequently the case that the date of death was only available for the husband. Consequently it was decided to modify the definition of "recently completed" so that in the event of divorce a family is included if the divorced husband/father had died between 1955 and 1970. This modification has negligible consequences for the subsequent analysis, since in the event of his not being the surviving parent, his ex-wife may also have died before 1970, but if not would only have

survived for more than a few years after that date in exceptional circumstances.

The data source is such that with few exceptions the entire sequence
of events (birth, marriages, divorces and deaths) can be established for
the whole family from the marriage of the parents through to the identifying death. As reported in the earlier paper the completeness of the data is
indicated by the fact that of the 603 families which had at least one child
and in which the parents did not divorce, only 24 had incomplete data.
The precise sequence is available because all events are dated to the day,
with the exception of divorce for which only the year is provided.

The source is the publication "Burke's Peerage." This lists the
descendents of the holders of British Peerages of the eighteenth century
(before that time family histories are considerably less complete). Nearly
half a million people are listed in order of descendency from past holders
of present titles. There may be reason to doubt the completeness of
certain aspects of the record. Some of the never married for example are
cited but not listed. In some instances dates for distant descendents
resident in other countries are not recorded. The requirement to allocate
each birth to a marriage will have undoubtedly misrepresented the sequence
of events in some instances. Nevertheless in the large majority of cases
the data appears to be complete and accurate (see: Bytheway 1974, for
checks against other sources).

The second aspect of this population which must be appreciated is
that, although it cannot be considered to be representative of Britain in
general, it does in fact constitute a complete population in itself. The fact
that a person is listed only because he is descended from a previous
holder means that every member of the population joined it at birth and
has remained so ever since. The only exception to this arises in the case
of extinct titles which are excluded from the 1970 volume. The bias that
this creates is discussed in Bytheway (1973). Because this bias is potentially important, it was decided to exclude all families that have contributed to the continuation of a title. In other words all 934 are the
families of younger brothers, cousins, etc. who have at no point inherited
the title under which they are listed. Inclusion is entirely independent of
any aspect of a family member's life such as length of life or number of
children (see: Bytheway, 1977a, for a discussion of the biasing effects
that such sampling procedures can have). Despite it being an autonomous
population, one wishes to argue that some generalization to Britain and
indeed contemporary western society is possible. Despite certain pecul-
iar cultural features of the British aristocracy, guarded generalisations

are indeed obviously possible, in much the same way, for example, as those that can be drawn from USA samples about the UK and vice versa.

It must be stressed that the 934 are a section of a real population rather than a simulated one and that its members have lived through a certain period of history. Of the fathers and sons of the 934 families 125 were reported as having died in the two World Wars. In the earlier paper I have argued that this does not invalidate the data—a comparable interplay with historical events will characterize any real population of families.

The median date of the 934 initial marriages is 1910; 90% occurred between 1890 and 1935. Most of the children, therefore will have been in their forties, fifties and sixties in 1970.

Complete Marital Careers

As reported in Bytheway (1979), 116 of the 934 marriages either ended in divorce or in a way that was not clear from the data—sometimes all that is known is that a person remarried. These 116 marriages were included as a consequence of the deaths of 91 husbands. Of these, the marital careers of 15 males, involving 22 divorced marriages, were incomplete in some way either because it was not clear how a marriage had ended or because a date of a marriage, divorce or death was missing.

The remaining 76 men had marital careers which included 158 marriages. By definition everyone of the 76 histories included one divorce. Of the other 82 marriages 19 also ended in divorce. Table 1 lists the frequencies of the different marital careers. This shows that although a simple history of marriage-divorce-second marriage is the most frequent sequence, it nevertheless characterizes only 33 careers; less than half of the whole sample.

Of these 33 completed marital careers of marriage-divorce-second marriage, the third and last phase—the second marriage—was the longest in 21 instances. This would conform with the assumption that divorce occurs earlier rather than later in life. In 12 of these 21 instances the man remarried in the same year or in the year following divorce, and of these 12, eight of the first marriages lasted between 7 and 12 years.

Thus by focusing at each division upon modal categories, we end up with an archetypical history: marriage of about ten years, divorce, remarriage within two years to the last the remainder of the man's life. Nevertheless this ''ideal'' or ''modal'' sequence characterizes only 8 out of 76 careers. Clearly the social scientist must be wary of his generalizations.

TABLE 1:   SEQUENCE OF EVENTS IN 76 MALE MARITAL HISTORIES

M = Marriage
D = Divorce
W = Death of wife

Sequence						Frequency
1st	2nd	3rd	4th	5th	6th	
M	D					13
M	D	M				33
M	D	M	D			3
M	D	M	W			7
M	W	M	D			1
M	D	M	D	M		11
M	D	M	W	M		2
M	W	M	D	M		2
M	D	M	D	M	D	1
M	D	M	D	M	W	1
M	D	M	W	M	D	1
M	W	M	D	M	D	1
				TOTAL		76

The Extended Family

Burke's Peerage, being based upon a patrilineal system of inheritance, records all descendents along male lines. The female offspring of male descendents are generally listed in full in the same way as the male (with the common exception that dates of birth may be omitted) but their children are only listed if the husbands were descendents themselves from a title. For this reason the full history of the extended family of each of the 76 "ego's" is available subject to the "extended family" being defined by diagram 1.

Although such a definition is unsatisfactory for many purposes, it is sufficiently detailed to provide some insight into the possible meanings of divorce within broader definitions of "family." This is obvious given the simple statistic that the average number of relatives (according to the above specification; excluding ego and all spouses of family members) is 22.5. The total numbers are shown in Table 2.

Within this definition of the extended family, what is the experience* of ego at different stages in his life regarding the subject of divorce?

---

*It is assumed that ego will become aware of changes in the marital status of each member of the extended family.

Table 3 presents the basic details. Of the 1709 relatives, 132 or 7.7% had been divorced at sometime prior to ego's death. Of the 132 "first divorces" of relatives, three occurred before ego was born, 25 before ego married and 58 before ego was himself divorced. This illustrates the obvious but important fact that the longer that ego lives, the more will be his experience of divorce within his family. This will be true irrespective of whether or not divorce "induces" or is statistically associated with further divorce within the family.

DIAGRAM 1:

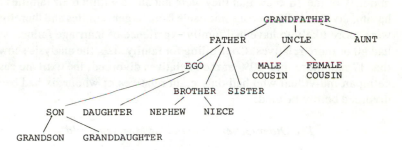

TABLE 2:   RELATIVES BORN BEFORE EGO'S DEATH

GRANDFATHERS	76
UNCLES	244
MALE COUSINS	240
FEMALE COUSINS	241
AUNTS	163
FATHERS	76
BROTHERS	128
NEPHEWS	72
NIECES	104
SISTERS	119
SONS	76*
GRANDSONS	45
GRANDDAUGHTERS	49
DAUGHTERS	76*
TOTAL	1709

* It is purely by a remarkable coincidence that the 76 males have between them 76 sons and 76 daughters.

Table 4 presents further detail about ego's relationships to the divorcees. Only 6 of the 76 had a father who had ever divorced and a further one whose grandfather had. In contrast 20 of the 152 offspring had divorced prior to their father's deaths. Most important, perhaps, is the fact that of their own generation, 9 siblings and 20 cousins were divorced prior to ego's own divorce.

Table 5 gives some idea of the extent to which individuals within the 76 had this kind of experience. Of the 76, 18 had at least one divorced relative by the time they married, 30 by the time they themselves were divorced and 50 within their lifetime. Thus by the time they died, the majority of the 76 knew that they were not alone within their families in having divorced. Of course some came from larger families and therefore were more likely to have had family experience of marriage failure: six had 40 or more relatives. Controlling for family size, the analysis shows that 17 had more than 20% of their relatives divorced, the extreme case being an individual who had only eight relatives of whom six had been divorced before he died.

The Older Generation and the Married Child

The above analysis relates to a cohort of males who have all died: their marital histories and experiences of divorce within a broad definition of the extended family. It is important that this overtime perspective of marital careers over the whole life span is fully appreciated. It should be stressed that this analysis has focused upon the marital career and extended family of the husband. Experience of divorce will obviously be more extensive within the joint family histories of a married couple. The longer a marriage survives the more probable it is that this experience will include more than just one divorce. It can be argued that such

TABLE 3:   EXPERIENCE OF MARRIAGE AND DIVORCE
IN EGO'S RELATIVES

	Total	Total ever Married	Total ever Divorced	Divorce Rate/1000
Ego's Birth	971	357	3	0.3
First Marriage	1318	691	25	1.9
First Divorce	1515	883	58	3.9
Death	1709	1125	132	7.7

TABLE 4: FREQUENCY OF EVER DIVORCED RELATIVES AT FOUR STAGES IN EGO'S LIFE

	Relatives divorced prior to:			
	Ego's Birth	First Marriage	First Divorce	Death
Grandfather	1			
Uncle		5	1	1
Male Cousin		7	13	11
Female Cousin		4	7	11
Aunt	1	1	2	
Father	1	3	1	1
Brother		1	6	10
Nephew				7
Niece				7
Sister		1	3	6
Son				8
Daughter				12
TOTAL	3	22	33	74

TABLE 5: NUMBER OF DIVORCED RELATIVES AT FOUR STAGES IN EGO'S LIFE

		Ego's Birth	First Marriage	First Divorce	Death
Number of Divorced Relatives	0	73	58	46	26
	1	3	12	13	13
	2		5	11	14
	3		1	3	10
	4			1	7
	5+			2	6
	TOTAL	76	76	76	76

personal experience will be an important source of knowledge in determining the character and consequences of a particular divorce process.

However, as indicated in the introduction and as may well be evident from other contributions to this monograph, much interest is centered upon the relationship between the divorcee and his or her parents. This particular data source can cast light upon the demographic aspects of this relationship from a slightly (but significantly) different perspective: the analysis begins not with a sample of divorces occurring within a population within a period of time, but rather with a sample of the older generation. The sample of 934 marriages has been introduced above with attention being focused upon 76 husbands who were divorced at some point in their lives. I now wish to return to the 934 couples and consider the extent to which the children of these marriages have married and divorced within the lifetimes of either or both of their parents. The 934 couples constitute a sample of the "older generation" with which we can examine the extent of their experience of child divorce. Of the 76 males, only 43 were divorced within the lifetimes of either or both parents and so in focusing attention upon the children of the 934 couples it is important to remember that a considerable number will divorce after both parents have died. In fact only 670 of the 934 couples had children, and of these only 594 had at least one child marry before the death of the surviving parent.* Our interest centers upon this period: that between the first marriage of a child (abbreviated to FMC) and the death of the surviving parent (abbreviated to DSP). What experience does the family have of child divorce: a family that has successfully reached the "childlaunching" stage?

Table 6 shows that these 594 families included 1473 children at the time of the FMC. There were 171 divorces within the lifetime of at least one parent. This table shows that divorce was most likely in the children of divorced parents. However we are not concerned in this paper to study such "pre-disposing" factors, but rather to describe the parental experience of child divorce. Parents divorced prior to FMC are a small and possibly "special" group. We do not have information about which household raised the children following divorce. Consequently we wish to focus attention upon the other two groups: those who were still married and those who were widowed at the FMC. Clearly with the married group we need to distinguish between the initial experience of the married couple and the later experience of the widow.** Table 7 gives an indication of the contrasting experiences of the three groups. Those people widowed before their FMC are fewest in number, but have proportionately the greatest experience of child divorce (23.2%). The

---

* As above, reference to the surviving parent is understood to imply the father if the parents had divorced.

** No distinction is made between the sexes in this analysis. Terms such as "widows" are used without such distinctions being implied.

other two groups are surprisingly similar, indicating that for these 360 families experience of divorce is fairly evenly divided by the event of widowhood.

This table is a little unfair to people who were widowed after their first child marriage. It implies that before and after bereavement are two distinct experiences. Table 8 combines them with those widowed before the first child marriage to illustrate the overall experience of child divorce of those who are or who become widows. Again this confirms generally assumed norms: that most parents do not experience any child divorce; and that of those that do, only a minority experience more than one.

If, however, we place divorce in the broader context of changes in

TABLE 6 : MARITAL STATUS OF PARENTS AT FMC

No. of	Married	Widowed*	Divorced*	
Families	360	194	40	594
Children	968	436	69	1473
Child Divorces	110	50	11	171
	11.1%	11.5%	15.9%	

* Including those who may have remarried

TABLE 7 : CHILD DIVORCE BETWEEN FMC AND DSP, BY PARENTAL MARITAL HISTORY AND NUMBER OF CHILDREN

		Surviving parent widowed before FMC			Period between FMC and first death			Period between first death and DSP		
No. of child divorces		0	1	2+	0	1	2+	0	1	2+
No. of children	1	58	9	1	67	9	0	73	5	0
	2	44	10	3	90	16	0	102	10	1
	3	31	12	0	85	12	1	78	13	3
	4+	16	10	0	65	13	2	55	11	2
TOTAL		149	41	4	307	50	3	308	39	6

(Both alive at FMC — spanning "Period between FMC and first death" and "Period between first death and DSP")

TABLE 8: CHILD DIVORCES BETWEEN FMC AND DSP EXPERIENCED SURVIVING PARENTS

		Number of child divorces prior to DSP				
		0	1	2	3	4
Number of children	1	121	21	2	0	0
	2	125	32	6	0	0
	3	102	35	2	1	1
	4	42	13	2	1	0
	5+	30	13	4	1	0
Total		420	114	16	3	1

marital status, then it becomes apparent that few parents have similar experiences. Table 9, for example, lists the different sequences experienced by the 45 marriages that produced two children of whom at least one divorced. Only 12 were characterised by the combined sequence of modal events: both children marrying and one divorcing and remarrying within the lifetime of the unremarried surviving parent.

Conclusion

Although this analysis could continue into much greater detail, the present purpose is simply to illustrate the experience that older people have of divorce. The analysis has separated their experiences of: (a) their own marital history, (b) divorce in a broadly defined extended family, and (c) divorce in the marriages of their own children.

This has shown that there are considerable variations between different families and that generalization about the experience of divorce over significant periods of life is difficult. If one assumes that personal experience of divorce, either in one's own marital career or in that of a member of the extended family, is an important aspect of the problem of understanding the divorce process—either for counselling or research purposes—then it is apparent that most people in this population will have had some such experience. Obviously this is more probable the older a person is, the greater his family or his range of acquaintances, and the higher the divorce rate within the population.

At the time of divorce itself there is of course only one divorce that "matters" and there are only four members of the older generation who count. Research that begins with divorce and then asks questions about the extended family is relatively straightforward. Clearly it is also extremely relevant to understanding more about the effect of divorce upon

TABLE 9:   FAMILIES OF TWO CHILDREN OF WHOM AT LEAST ONE DIVORCED:
SEQUENCE OF EVENTS BETWEEN FMC AND DSP

PARENTAL STATE AT FMC	SEQUENCE OF EVENTS (INC. FMC)	PARENTAL STATE AT FMC	SEQUENCE OF EVENTS (INC. FMC)
UNREMARRIED WIDOW(ER)	1 M M V	BOTH ALIVE AND MARRIED	21 M B M V M
	2 M M V M		22 M B M V M
	3 M M V M		23 M B M V M
	4 M M V M		24 M B V M
	5 M M V M W		25 M M B R V M
	6 M M W V M M		26 M M B V
	7 M V M M		27 M M B V M
	8 M V M R M D V M B		28 M M B V V
			29 M M B W V
REMARRIED WIDOW(ER)	9 M M V M B		30 M M C V
	10 M M V V M M		31 M M D V M D B
	11 M M W V M M		32 M M V B
	12 M V M B X		33 M M V B M
	13 M V M V M B W M M		34 M M V B R V
			35 M M V B W
DIVORCED: FATHER REMARRIED*	14 M M V M B		36 M M V M B
	15 M M V M V M B		37 M M V M B
	16 M M V M W M		38 M M V M B
	17 M V M B R X		39 M M V M B D D
	18 M V M M		40 M M V M B V M
	19 M V M X		41 M M W V M D B
	20 M V X		42 M V B M
			43 M V M B W X
			44 M V M B X
			45 M V M D B

* There were no cases in this series of a divorced father not having remarried before FMC.

KEY TO SYMBOLS:

	CHILD	PARENT*
Marriage	M	R
Widowhood	W	B
Divorce	V	C
Death	D	
Alive at DSP and never married	X	

* For families 14-20 these symbols refer only to the father.

family relationships. It is also important, however, to conduct research which begins with the extended family and then asks questions about divorce. The fact that this analysis has shown that demographically this is no simple task does not reduce the importance of this perspective.

It may be a statistical fact that women do tend to divorce shortly after their fathers die, or that fathers tend to die shortly after their daughters divorce, or that similar relationships exist between mothers and sons, or that children tend to divorce shortly after their parents divorce, or that parents divorce shortly after their children marry. If any such statistical relationship exists, then it follows that divorce cannot be assumed to be simply the failure of an isolated phenomenon: the marriage of two individuals. It is important that research is instigated that looks at marriage and divorce from this wider perspective and is not restricted by normative beliefs about the true course of family life.

REFERENCES

BYTHEWAY, W. R.

Sampling biases and familial units, University of Keele, SRUS Occasional Paper No. 3, 1973.

"The Dynamics of Family Structures", Ph.D. Thesis, University of Keele, 1974.

Problems of Representation in "The Three Generation Family Study", *Journal of Marriage and Family Living*, *39*, pp 239-250, 1977a.

Aspects of Old Age in Age-Specific Mortality Rates, (originally published in *Journal of Biosocial Science*, 2, 1970), in: Death and Society: A Book of Readings and Sources, (Eds. Carse, James and Dallery, Arleen, Harcourt Brace Jovanovich, pp 313-326, 1977b.

Ageing and Sociological Studies of the Family, in: Family Life in Old Age (Eds. Dooghe, G. and Helander, J.), Martinus Nijhoff, The Hague, pp 15-22, 1979.

THE ROLE OF EXTENDED KIN IN THE
ADJUSTMENT TO MARITAL SEPARATION

Graham B. Spanier
Sandra Hanson

ABSTRACT. A nonprobability purposive sample of 205 individuals separated 26 months or less was interviewed about their marital separation and its aftermath. Contrary to expectations based on earlier research and current theorizing, the findings indicate that support from and interaction with extended kin either are unrelated or negatively related to the adjustment to marital separation. The findings further suggest that the potential advantages of support and interaction offered by kin may be moderated by a variety of familial sanctions such as criticism and disapproval. These results, however, replicated Goode's (1956) finding from an earlier generation, which demonstrated that adjustment was enhanced when kin were indifferent to the divorce—neither offering approval nor disapproval. The results also suggest that in many cases it is likely that adjustment to separation begins before the time relatives first learn of the separation.

Introduction

The complexity and difficulty of adjustment to marital separation and the vast numbers of people who are involved in the process suggest a real need for theoretical and empirical knowledge in this area. The upward

Graham B. Spanier, PhD, is Associate Professor of Human Development and Sociology, Department of Individual and Family Studies, The Pennsylvania State University, University Park, PA. 16802. Sandra Hanson, PhD, is an Assistant Professor in the Department of Sociology, University of Missouri, St. Louis, MO 63121. This is a revision of a paper presented at the annual meeting of the Southern Sociological Society, New Orleans, March, 1978. Research for this paper was supported by grant R03MH 27706 of the National Institute of Mental Health.

trend in the rate of divorce which began in the early 1960's has promoted considerable interest in the various factors causing divorce. However, the social-psychological adjustment of the separated person has received very little attention (Rose, & Price-Bonham, 1973; Freund, 1974).

This paper explores the role of extended kin in post-separation adjustment. It tests hypotheses that two independent variables, involvement with extended kin and support from extended kin, positively influence the quality of adjustment experienced in the post-separation period. The hypotheses were tested with cross-sectional data from face-to-face structured interviews conducted with a non-probability purposive sample of 205 recently separated people in Central Pennsylvania.

Following Weiss (1975), the research design called for separation rather than divorce as the primary criterion for sampling. An assumption of the study was that separation was the more critical social-psychological event for the persons involved. Furthermore, due to Pennsylvania's adversary system of divorce law and the possibility of legal maneuvering on issues of child custody, support, visitation, and property settlements, divorce is often delayed considerably beyond the time of physical, emotional, financial, or social-psychological separation. In our sample, 76 percent of the recently separated respondents were already divorced by the time of the interview. Twenty four percent were separated but not yet divorced.

The Role of Extended Kin in the Adjustment to Separation

There is a trend in family life toward less interaction with co-workers and neighbors due to the depersonalization which accompanies urban and industrial life. Consequently, there is a greater reliance on and interaction with kin (Bell & Boat, 1957; Greer, 1954; Dotson, 1956; Reiss, 1962; Sussman & Burchinal, 1962; Leichter & Mitchell, 1967; Adams, 1968). The literature suggests that kin are relied upon more than any other group for services, aid, and in emergencies (Bell & Boat, 1957; Axelrod, 1956). Assistance in times of need is a crucial binding factor in social relationships and it has been shown that kin provide much of the assistance at these times (Leichter & Mitchell, 1969).

A review of previous literature on separation and divorce indicates that kin play a vital role in the process of adjustment to separation. One of the variables with which our research is concerned—the receipt of support—has been singled out by several authors as being valuable for the separated person's adjustment. Kin often prove helpful by making their homes available, offering services such as child care, providing companionship, and lending money (Weiss, 1975). Separated individuals end up receiving economic and emotional support from extended kin even though there are no institutionalized norms delineating the direction and degree of obligation (Goode, 1956). This support might allow the individual to continue to play necessary roles and fulfill ordinary obligations at work and in the community. Support then, satisfies certain needs in the new role situation and as a result, is important for good adjustment (Goode, 1956; Freund, 1974; Weiss, 1975). One can predict that support typically will come from kin during the adjustment process and that this source of support will lead to better adjustment, because of the intimate and customarily supportive nature of the interaction. In addition, it is likely that support from extended kin does not involve some of the burdensome obligations of support from other sources. For example, interest may not be charged for monetary loans. Furthermore, kin support may be superior to support from friends, co-workers, or commercial establishments because of the absence of a feeling of obligation to return aid after receiving it.

The second factor which has been thought to enhance adjustment is social interaction. Adequate social interaction following divorce has been found to be critical in reducing stress (Raschke, 1974; Goode, 1956). Presumably, by keeping active in the new role, the person is defined by others and consequently sees himself or herself as an adequately functioning individual who commands some respect in the new status and who is able to perform in day-to-day social roles. Social interaction and the resultant redefinition by self and others of the new status hastens the modification of self concept which adjustment involves.

It is important to note that although research shows that family members usually end up supporting and interacting with a separated person, this may not always be the case, and some writers have suggested that the separation or divorce of a relative may result in noteworthy exceptions to the rule (Levinger, 1966; Bohannon, 1971; Wheeler, 1974; Burgess, Locke, & Thomas, 1971). Kin may not know how to handle the separation and thus may hesitate to become involved (Freund, 1974; Bohannon, 1971). They may even take sides (Burgess, Locke, & Thomes, 1971) or act in unpredictable ways (Lasswell & Lasswell, 1973). In addition, even if kin do lend support and interact with a separated relative, they may place a certain amount of stigma on the individual undergoing separation.

Hypotheses

Evidence suggests that sociability varies in quality, and consequently varies in its ability to fulfill needs for persons (Weiss, 1975). Social relationships with extended kin may have a more positive effect on satisfaction with life than other social relationships. The typically comfortable and intimate social settings surrounding kinship relations presumably are likely to produce interaction conducive to more positive social-psychological adjustment. We are thus able to formulate two hypotheses:

1. The greater the number of relatives providing support following marital separation, the better the individual's adjustment to separation.
2. The more social interaction the separated person has with extended kin following marital separation, the better the individual's adjustment to separation.

Positive adjustment to separation involves regaining individual autonomy following a marital separation. Broadly defined, the term can be conceptualized as a process whereby "a disruption of role sets and patterns, or existing social relations, is incorporated into the individual's life pattern, such that the roles accepted and assigned do not take the prior divorce into account as the primary point of reference" (Goode, 1956:19). The independent variable, social interaction, is used to denote any sort of direct contact with individuals or participation in groups of individuals. The concept "support" includes help given to the separated person. This help may consist of lending or giving money, offering services such as babysitting or home repair, and giving moral support.

Sampling and Data Collection

The data, collected during the Spring of 1977, consisted of in-depth, structured, face-to-face interviews focusing on the social, psychological, and economic adjustments of males and females who had experienced a marital separation within the preceeding 26 months, whether or not they were divorced. The larger project of which this paper is a part made use of two techniques: analysis of case histories through in-depth, unstructured interviewing techniques, and survey research using structured questionnaire schedules. Non-probability, purposive sampling techniques were used in the second phase of the research. The population from which the sample was drawn consisted of all those separated persons in Centre County, Pennsylvania whose separation had taken place since January, 1975.

The location and selection of individuals was accomplished through various methods. Newspaper articles describing the project and generally discussing divorce were placed in several local newspapers. The purpose of these articles was to alert the community to the study, and to attempt to set a tone for the study which might elicit cooperation and a better response rate than is customary for research in this area. This strategy proved to be the most helpful technique for increasing our response rate, since most of our respondents had read about the study and "felt it was legitimate" after learning about it from the newspaper. Additionally, a few people responded to these articles by volunteering for the study. Letters were sent to all attorneys in the county informing them of the study, and the domestic relations office staff was contacted for cooperation. These contacts also produced a few respondents.

The main tool for obtaining participants involved the procurement from public documents in the county courthouse of names and addresses of those who had recently separated or divorced. A team from the project abstracted the files of eligible persons. Eligible respondents included persons still living within 50 miles of the county who had either: (1) filed for divorce, but had not yet received a decree, (2) obtained a divorce decree, or (3) separated and filed (or were filed against) for custody or support. Individuals who were informally separated, but had not sought custody or support, were obtained by the forms of solicitation mentioned above and additionally, through snowball sampling techniques.

Letters were then sent to possible participants describing the study and requesting a response. We were able to identify 918 eligible respondents in the county. After three follow up letters and numerous attempts via telephone to contact persons directly, we were able to make contact with 344, or 37 percent, of the eligible respondents. Two hundred ten, or 61 percent, of these persons agreed to be interviewed, and actually completed the interview. These low response rates are consistent with those obtained in similar recent studies. This high degree of self-selection in our sample undoubtedly reduces heterogeneity in the study, but it is not known how those who participated differed from those who did not. Five interviews were discarded after it was determined that these persons had been separated for longer than 26 months. Interviews ranged from one and one-half to three hours, with a mean length of two hours and fifteen minutes. The interview schedule contained approximately 550 questions.

Measurement

One independent variable, support from extended kin, was operationalized through a combined index of three questions asking which persons had helped with service, finances, and moral support since the separation. A list of alternatives was given, including friends, coworkers, and an exhaustive range of extended kin. Individual scores on this index were obtained by adding up the number of kin listed as giving support. All types of support were weighed equally. Thus, the individual's final score on this index represented the number of kin who had helped in service, financial, and moral areas.

The other independent variable, interaction with extended kin, was operationalized through the use of a question which asked the respondent to list the three persons closest to him or her, to specify whether they were kin or nonkin, and to specify how often the respondent had contact with these persons. Concerning frequency of contact, a list of frequencies was given with alternatives ranging from "daily" to "never." Individual scores for this variable were obtained by adding up frequencies of contact with the closest persons who were listed as kin. The greater the amount of interaction an individual had with extended kin, the higher his or her score would be on this variable.

The dependent variable, adjustment to separation, was operationalized by using four separate adjustment scales. The first measures satisfaction with life. The item asked, "Now we'd like to know how satisfied you are with certain things in your day-to-day life. Please pick the choice which best describes how satisfied you are with [then listed sequentially] the work you do, where you live, your way of life, the things you do for enjoyment, and your health." The choices consisted of "extremely satisfied," "somewhat satisfied," and "not satisfied." Cronbach's alpha reliability for this scale was .71 in our sample.

A second adjustment scale, adapted from Rosenberg (1965), measured self-esteem. Persons were asked in this question to state the extent to which they agreed or disagreed with a number of items such as "I feel I have a number of good qualities." Cronbach's alpha reliability for the scale was .87 in our sample.

The third index of adjustment was adapted from Bradburn and Caplovitz (1965). It measures a variety of positive and negative feelings along with the frequency of their occurrence. For example, respondents were asked how often during the past week they felt "particularly excited or interested in something." Responses ranged from "never" to "often." Cronbach's alpha reliability for this scale was .77 in our sample.

Finally, adjustment to separation was measured by an index adapted from Kitson and Sussman (1974), which specifically dealt with the separation. Respondents were asked to state the extent to which certain statements such as "Sometimes I can't believe we got a divorce (separation)." and "I'm angry at my (former) spouse." expressed their feelings. Alternatives to these statements ranged from "Not at all" to "Very much." Cronbach's alpha reliability for this scale was .85 in our sample.

Methodological Issues and Limitations

This study has certain limitations which restrict one's ability to generalize the findings to other populations and situations. Since a nonprobability sampling technique was used, the sample may contain noteworthy biases. The sample was small and was selected from a mostly white population within a largely rural Pennsylvania county. Another limitation concerns the high refusal rate experienced in the study. Only 61 percent of those contacted participated and there is no way of knowing the social-psychological characteristics of those who we could not contact or who refused to participate.

The operationalization of kin interaction used in the study depended on amount of interaction only, not on quality of interaction. Since quality of interaction may be just as important, if not more important, than amount of interaction, future researchers might want to include both quality and frequency in their operationalization of interaction.

Selected Characteristics of the Sample

Ages of the respondents varied from 20 to 67 with a mean age of 33 and standard deviation of 8.9. Forty-four percent (N = 91) of the sample was male and 56 percent was female (N = 114). The total yearly income was less than $5,000 for 28 percent of the sample. Thirty one percent of the sample had a total yearly income between $5,000 and $9,999, while 23 percent had an income range of $10,000 and $14,999. The remainder of the respondents, 18 percent, had incomes greater than $15,000. A majority of the individuals in the sample had at least a few relatives living within a one hour drive. Forty three percent had no immediate relatives living within a one hour drive and 41 percent had none of their spouses' relatives living within a one hour drive. The sample was 12 percent Roman Catholic and 60 percent Protestant. Nine percent stated other religious preferences, and 19 percent were atheist, agnostic, or had no religious preference.

Table 1. Percent Reporting Receipt of Moral, Financial, and Service Support From Selected Sources for Men (and Women)

Source of Support	TYPE OF SUPPORT*		
	Moral	Financial	Service
Mother	86.1 (90.3)	18.8 (52.4)	35.4 (48.1)
Father	70.8 (83.9)	27.0 (49.4)	35.2 (50.6)
Brothers, Sisters	73.3 (83.0)	11.4 (18.9)	29.9 (50.9)
Mother-in-Law	20.7 (30.0)	2.4 (9.0)	9.6 (14.4)
Father-in-Law	23.0 (19.3)	2.6 (5.8)	8.1 (12.4)
Brothers, Sisters-in-Law	30.9 (34.6)	0.0 (1.8)	6.1 (20.2)
Co-workers	71.1 (80.8)	4.4 (1.9)	30.0 (76.3)
Friends	84.6 (95.6)	6.6 (32.5)	54.9 (73.0)

*Percentages total more than 100 since respondents typically reported multiple sources of support. Percentages for women are listed after percentages for men.

Nature and Extent of Kinship Support and Interaction

Table 1 summarizes separately for men and women the sources of kinship and other support reported by our respondents. Our separated respondents appear to rely on parents and siblings for moral support as well as on friends and work associates. With regard to financial help, persons rely primarily on parents and rarely on other kin. Service support also is provided by parents and siblings, as well as friends and work associates. In all but two instances, women receive more support than do men. It is interesting to note that women report receiving more service and moral support from their co-workers than do men. A picture of fairly extensive kin support emerges from these data, although it is clear that friends and co-workers also play a significant part in support of individuals who are adjusting to a separation.

When asked about their parents' reaction to their separation, 64 percent of the sample stated that their parents pretty much stayed out of it. Twenty three percent had parents who encouraged them to go through with it, and 12 percent had parents who encouraged them not to go through with it. More in-laws (44 percent) than parents (36 percent) were reported to have become involved by encouraging or discouraging the separation.

Descriptive data on the nature and extent of support from and interaction with extended kin were obtained. Females receive more support from their kin than males in services provided ($\chi^2 = 15.4$, df = 6, p < .01) and financial help ($\chi^2 = 21.0$, df = 6, p < .001). There were no significant differences between the genders in moral support from kin ($\chi^2 = 7.8$, df = 6, N.S.). Likewise, there was no significant relationship between gender and amount of interaction with kin ($\chi^2 = .01$, df = 1, N.S.).

There were no differences found in amount of moral support, financial support, or help with services between those who were separated but not yet divorced and those who were divorced. In addition, there were no differences in kinship interaction between the separated and divorced.

The initial impression one gets from our data is that kin, especially parents, play an important role in post-separation adjustment. Other data lend additional support to this notion. One half of the sample listed a relative as a person closest to them during the last year or two of marriage, and 43 percent listed a relative as the person closest to them now. In addition, 46 percent and 32 percent of the sample, respectively, listed relatives as the second and third closest persons to them at the time of the interview.

Despite this rather consistent picture of kin support and interaction during this difficult time of crisis for most of our respondents, a different picture of the role of kin in the adjustment to separation emerged when we tested our hypotheses. Zero-order Pearsonian correlations were obtained for the relationships between our independent variables (support from and interaction with extended kin) and our dependent adjustment variables. These correlations are presented in Table 2. One significant relationship was discovered between interaction with kin and adjustment, and one significant relationship was found between support from kin and adjustment. There were negative relationships between support from kin and adjustment to separation, and interaction with kin and adjustment to separation, as measured by a scale asking about feelings concerning the former spouse and marriage.

In order to discover whether the absence of significant relationships was due to one or more suppressor variables (Rosenberg, 1968), partial correlations were obtained, controlling for length of separation, proximity to kin, and sex. This analysis indicated that none of the test factors were acting as suppressor variables. Thus, the lack of confirmation for the hypotheses additionally was supported by the partial correlation analysis.

The hypotheses were also tested by regressing the adjustment variables on amount of interaction with kin and support from kin. None of the variables in the regression analysis were significant at the .05 level. Neither interaction with kin nor support from kin explain a significant amount of variance in adjustment, as measured by the feelings, self esteem, satisfaction, and adjustment to separation scales. It is interesting to note, however, that a majority of the regression coefficients were negative.

A second set of regression analyses were performed, controlling for several variables which might potentially have a supressing effect on the original relationships between the independent variables and the adjustment variables. The variables which were included as controls in these regressions were: sex, length of separation, number of children, proximity to kin, income, and age. Once again, the regression coefficients for interaction with kin and support from kin were not significant at the .05 level in any of the regression equations.

Although kin support in general was not related to adjustment in this sample, we were interested in discovering whether specific types of support might affect adjustment to separation. Three support indexes were created in the areas of moral, financial, and service help. Regres-

Table 2. Pearsonian Correlations Between Interaction with Kin, Support from Kin and Four Measures of Adjustment

	Positive/Negative Feelings Scale	Self Esteem Scale	Satisfaction with Life Scale	Adjustment to Separation Scale
Kin Support	- .04	- .05	- .01	- .16*
Kin Interaction	- .08	- .08	- .08	- .15*

*Significant at .05 level

sion analyses were then performed with these indexes. None of the independent variables in this analysis involving the support indexes were significant at the .05 level. In addition to looking at the effect of various types of support or adjustment, the effect of different sources of support is of interest. Since researchers have discovered that of various kin, parents especially may feel free to criticize and evaluate their children's activities, it is possible that those who get greater amounts of support from siblings than from parents may fare better in the adjustment process. Our sample was classified according to those who received a greater amount of support from parents than from siblings, and to those who received a greater amount of support from siblings than from parents. Adjustment was then assessed in a regression evaluating support for each of these groups. One significant regression relation appeared— for the group who had greater support from parents than from siblings. This relation was negative in direction and was significant at the .01 level. This finding supports the hypothesis that parental support may be accompanied by negative evaluation or condemnation, thus detracting from adjustment to separation. The data from this study did not allow for an investigation of the differential effects of kin and nonkin support (i.e., friends, coworkers). Other researchers might be interested in looking at these relationships.

A problem that is frequently encountered in the investigation of relationships is that of causal order. One might argue that quality of adjustment affects the amount of support and interaction received rather than vice versa. For example, it is possible that kin may lend more support due to the fact that an individual is experiencing a poor adjustment. The adjustment measure which we chose to look at with respect to this relationship was that of financial loss or financial neediness. The variable was constructed by comparing the respondent's financial situation before and after separation. If a person's post-separation economic stability was reported to be worse than his or her pre-separation economic stability, he or she was categorized as having experienced a loss of financial or economic stability. The interaction between financial/economic loss and support was examined and was not found to be significant in an additional regression. This finding suggests that persons experiencing different degrees of financial/economic loss do not receive different amounts of support from kin.

In this study, two types of kin-oriented activity—support and interaction—were found to have no effect on adjustment to separation. It is enlightening to look at how these same types of activities affect adjustment when they are friend-oriented. Individual scores for an interaction with friends variable were obtained by adding frequencies of contact with the closest persons who were listed as friends. The adjustment to separation scale score was regressed on the interaction with friends variable, with sex, age, income, and length of separation included as controls. Interaction with friends was found to be significant in this regression at the .01 level. Thus, interaction with friends was found in this sample to contribute positively to adjustment. Consequently, this finding poses an additional question of interest: How is interaction with kin related to interaction with friends, and does the relationship between these two variables affect the relationship between interaction with kin and adjustment to marital separation? It is possible that those with considerable involvement with kin seek kin for support because they have few friends. Likewise, those who interact often with friends may not interact with their kin very often. If these two interaction variables are negatively related, one might expect the inclusion of the interaction with friend variable in a regression equation involving the kin and adjustment variables to change the predictability of the relationship between interaction with kin and adjustment to separation.

The variables interaction with kin and interaction with friends are correlated $-.87$, using a Pearsonian correlation, significant at the .001 level. The inclusion of the interaction with friends variable in the regression equation changed the interaction with kin predictor from a negative to a positive value, and increased its magnitude. However, the statistic was still not significant at the .05 level. It appears, then, that when one considers that some persons have more interaction with friends than others, and concomitantly less interaction with kin than others, the relationship between interaction with kin and adjustment to separation becomes positive, but is not significant.

Discussion

Previous theory and research on extended kin relations and marital dissolution led to the prediction that kin interaction and support are variables which contribute to better adjustment to marital separation. The findings from this research do not support that prediction. The sample studied had a high incidence of interaction with and support from kin, yet adjustment is either not contingent on or negatively related to these variables. There are several critical factors pertaining to kin interaction which may help explain the finding.

The decision to separate usually is reached over an extended period of time. Some adjustment relative to the separation may actually occur before the separation occurs. It has been stated that in many nuclear families, there is a desire to be close—but not too close—to extended kin. Many marital problems, then, may never be reported to relatives (Weiss, 1975). It is possible that kin are unaware of marital problems at the critical time when separation is being discussed, seriously considered, and implemented. Thus, relatives may be unable to give support at a critical time, and consequently may have little influence in an adjustment process which is already underway.

Presence or absence of familial approval or disapproval of a separation was found by Goode (1956) to relate to adjustment. In his sample, 60 percent of the respondents' families approved, and 20 percent disapproved, of the separation. Respondents in Goode's sample were less likely to say that friends had approved or disapproved. According to Goode, when there is high approval or disapproval, the involvement of kin in the conflict is likely to be great. The most favorable situation for low trauma, he states, is one in which major reference groups are viewed by the individual as being relatively indifferent to the divorce. The highest proportion of high trauma cases was found by Goode when various groups actively disapproved of the divorce or separation.

Relatives, especially parents, may sometimes feel that their commitment (or bond) to the separated person obligates them to evaluate the decision to separate. Parents especially may feel they are free to comment on the separation, to criticize it, and to disapprove or approve of it (Weiss, 1975). Parents may feel that a marriage has been ended frivolously and may urge reconciliation. They may find it hard to understand the concept of "incompatability" and may argue for "trying harder." Parents and siblings may somehow feel they are to blame for the breakup. A recurrent complaint in Weiss's (1975) sample of divorced persons was that separated individuals wanted to be treated with acceptance, but they did not want intrusion. On the other hand, parents want to know and understand all that has gone wrong.

Kin, then, by virtue of their special status and the emotional investment they may have in the marriage, may react to the separation or divorce situation in a way which would hinder, rather than help, adjustment. Apparently, the interaction and especially the support which kin offer may be tempered by evaluation, disapproval, criticism, and other intrusions which they feel free to voice.

Although separation, and subsequently divorce, is a common phenomenon in American society, it is possible that there continues to be a lack of institutionalized norms for dealing with it. Because of the resulting inability of the kinship structure to provide unambiguous arrangements in areas of support and interaction, and the lack of prescriptions regarding reaction to marital separation, an ambiguous situation may be created whereby adjustment to separation becomes difficult. The ambiguities may center around when and how to give financial, moral, and service support. A further point of ambiguity may involve the redefinition of individuals with regard to their former kinship structure. Goode (1956) points out that our society is typified by an emphasis on the family unit. This situation may leave some separated persons virtually on their own.

A majority of the parents of our respondents belong to the generational cohort of people who were born in the early 1900's. Many in this cohort can be characterized as having an orientation which does not favor divorce. A divorce in the family may be a traumatic, even disgracing, event. While support may be forthcoming, it may be difficult to offer, and negative evaluation can come easily.

It is possible that the families in which high interaction is the norm are the more traditional families with the most negative attitudes toward divorce. It is also possible that individuals who belong to these traditional families have the least autonomy from the family and so are more affected by any negative evaluation which might be directed toward them.

Conclusions

It is apparent that more research in the area of adjustment to separation is needed. Separation and subsequent divorce are complex events and many variables interact to influence adjustment. Factors such as social relationships, financial stress, the legal system, attitudes of family and community toward separation, and remarriage are theoretically important variables which are being examined in other reports from the current study.

Support from extended kin and interaction with extended kin were found in this research to be unrelated to three measures of adjustment. A great majority of the sample received significant amounts of support and interaction from kin, but these variables are not predictive of adjustment. While kin often offer a variety of unwanted evaluations and criticisms which may create additional stress, the support and interaction they offer is not matched by any other group of people. Those without kin support may go supportless. Nevertheless, our data lead us to the conclusion that the customarily positive influences of kinship relationships do not help the recently separated individual with important social-psychological adjustments. Although support is forthcoming, it seems to do little to enhance adjustment. As new cohorts of parents and relatives emerge, and as divorce becomes a more institutionalized and accepted phenomenon, familial reaction to divorce may become less burdensome for the separated person, and future researchers might expect to find a more positive relationship between the variables examined.

REFERENCES

Adams, B. *Kinship in an urban setting*. Chicago: Markham, 1968.
Axelrod, M. Urban structure and social participation. *American Sociological Review*, 1956, *21*, 13-18.
Bell, W., & Boat, M. D. Urban neighborhoods and informal social relations. *American Journal of Sociology*, 1957, *62*, 391-398.
Bohannan, P. Some thoughts on divorce reform. In P. Bohannan (Ed.), *Divorce and after*. New York: Doubleday, 1971.
Bradburn, M., & Caplovitz, D. *Reports on happiness*. Chicago: University of Chicago Press, 1965.
Burgess, E. W., Locke, J., & Thomes, M. M. *The family* (4th ed.). New York: Van ostrand Reinhold, 1971.
Dotson, F. Patterns of voluntary association among working class families. *American Sociological Review*, 1951, *61*, 687-693.
Freund, J. Divorce and grief. *Journal of Family Counseling*, 1974, *2*, 40-43.
Goode, W. J. *After divorce*. Glencoe, Ill.: Free Press, 1956.
Greer, S. Urbanism reconsidered: A comparative study of local areas in a metropolis. *American Sociological Review*, 1956, *21*, 19-25.
Kitson, G. & Sussman, M. Unpublished interview schedule, Case Western Reserve University, Cleveland, Ohio, 1976.
Lasswell, M. E., & Lasswell, T. E. *Love, marriage, family: A developmental approach. Introduction to part 13*. Glenview, Ill.: Scott, Foresman, 1973.
Leichter, H. J., & Mitchell, W. E. *Kinship and case work*. Hartford: Communication Printers, Inc., 1967.
Levinger, G. Sources of marital dissatisfaction among applicants for divorce. *Journal of Orthopsychiatry*, 1966, *36*, 803-807.
Raschke, H. J. Social and psychological factors in post-marital dissolution adjustment. Doctoral dissertation, University of Minnesota, 1974.
Reiss, P. J. Extended kinship system: Correlates of and attitudes on frequency of interaction. *Journal of Marriage and the Family*, 1962, *24*, 333-340.
Rose, V. L., & Price-Bonham, S. Divorce adjustment: A woman's problem? *Family Coordinator*, 1973, *22*, 291-297.
Rosenberg, M. *Society and the adolescent self image*. Princeton, New Jersey: Princeton University Press, 1965.
Rosenberg, M. *The logic of survey analysis*. New York: Basic Books, 1968.
Sussman, M., & Burchinal, L. Kin family network: Unheralded structure in current conceptualization of family functioning. *Marriage and Family Living*, 1962, *24*, 231-240.
Weiss, R. S. *Marital separation*. New York: Basic Books, 1975.
Wheeler, M. *No-fault divorce*. Boston: Beacon Press, 1974.

CHANGES IN FAMILY RELATIONSHIPS
FOLLOWING DIVORCE OF ADULT CHILD:
GRANDMOTHER'S PERCEPTIONS

Constance R. Ahrons
Madonna E. Bowman

ABSTRACT. This paper presents findings from interviews with 78 grandmothers whose son or daughter experienced a divorce. Grandmothers were questioned regarding the effects of divorce on their relationships with their divorced child, their former in-law, and their grandchildren. Respondents' feelings about their child's divorce were also explored. Overall, mothers appeared to provide support to their divorced child and relatively few felt the divorce had a negative impact on their own lives. Implications of legally protecting the grandparent-grandchild relationship are examined.

Relatively little attention has been paid to the effects of divorce on intergenerational family relationships. The scarcity of research on family processes of the divorced family results in part from the fact that the postdivorce family has no historical precedent in western society (Bohannan, 1971; Mead, 1971). However, the dramatic increase in divorce rates

Constance R. Ahrons, PhD, is Associate Professor of Social Work, and Madonna E. Bowman, MSSW is a PhD candidate in Social Welfare, University of Wisconsin, Madison. This research was supported in part by HEW-AoA Grant #90-A-1230 for multidisciplinary research on Aging Women, awarded to the Faye McBeath Institute on Aging and Adult Life, University of Wisconsin-Madison (1977–1979).

49

indicates that divorced families will make up a large part of this country's family life in the next decade. Although several recent longitudinal studies have explored the reorganization of the nuclear family following divorce, these studies have not included members of the extended families (Ahrons, 1979, 1980b; Hetherington, Cox and Cox, 1976; Wallerstein and Kelly, 1979).

The process of divorce, conceptualized as a crisis of family transition and change, requires major familial reorganization (Ahrons, 1980a, 1980c). Bohannan (1971) has identified the complex patterns of family reorganization that results from divorce chains (relationships formed among spouses and ex-spouses). Furstenburg (1979) elaborated on Bohannan's work by exploring the impact of remarriage on kinship configurations, noting that "remarriage chains" might better describe the process of "family recycling" that is evolving. Ahrons (1979, 1980a, 1981) has found that some divorced families are reorganizing into binuclear families—families with two households of orientation. Common to all these frameworks is the fact that increased divorce rates have resulted in new, complex family networks with altered kinship systems. Research, while focusing on the child's adjustment to the marital disruption, has only been concerned peripherally with the impact on relationships within the family system.

To date, the limited information available on the impact of divorce on intergenerational family relationships has been obtained from the middle, divorced generation. The research indicates consensus that contact between first and second generation affines (in-laws) is substantially reduced following divorce (Spicer and Hampe, 1975; Anspach, 1976). Gongla and Wales, who studied the impact of divorce on only those relationships which women identified as most significant prior to marital separation, found that relationships with affines were more likely to suffer than relationships with consanguines (blood kin). There is also evidence which indicates that relationships of first and second generation consanguines may even become somewhat closer following divorce. Anspach (1976) found that two-thirds of the remarried and one-third of the currently divorced women in his sample reported increased contact with consanguines following divorce. Similarly, Spicer and Hampe (1975) reported 18.3% of their respondents indicated increased contact with consanguines after divorce. However, Gongla and Wales found that relationships with consanguines were likely to remain unchanged following divorce. If change did occur it was likely to reflect improvement in the relationship. Evidence regarding changes in men's contact with consanguines following divorce is very limited. Spicer and Hampe (1975) found only 13% of men reported increased contact with consanguines following divorce while 26% of women indicated increased contact.

These findings, the attenuation of relationships between affines and stability of relationships between consanguines following divorce, have implications for both the first (grandparent) and third (grandchild) generations. It has been suggested that parents mediate the relationships between their own parents and their children (Kennedy and Pfeifer, 1973; Robertson, 1975). Therefore, it would follow that when divorce reduces contact of the middle generation with either the first or third generation it would also be expected to alter the relationship of the grandparent and grandchild generations. As noted earlier, evidence regarding changes in men's contact with consanguines following divorce is quite limited. We do know, however, that men are typically noncustodial parents following divorce and that their access to their children is markedly lower than during marriage. Thus we would hypothesize that contact between paternal grandparents and their grandchildren would decline following divorce, and that the contact with maternal grandparents should remain unchanged or perhaps increase. Anspach's (1976) data support both the parent as mediator theory, and the hypothesis that paternal grandparents are more likely to lose contact with grandchildren following divorce than are maternal grandparents.

A recent change in the Wisconsin divorce law reflects this concern for the kinship relationship between first and third generations. While intergenerational family ties (other than between parents and minor children) have not been a central concern in family policy, the 1978 revision of Wisconsin divorce statutes legally recognizes the rights of grandparents in divorced family systems. The statute allows grandparents to petition the court for visitation of grandchildren whose parents are divorced. This provision may have far reaching implications for intergenerational family relationships.

The impact of divorce on intergenerational family relationships provides the major focus of the present investigation. This study is unique in that it was based on the perceptions of the first or grandparent generation rather than the middle generation and includes data from mothers of both divorced sons and divorced daughters. Three major questions were addressed in this study:

1. How does divorce affect intergenerational family relationships? Specifically, how does it affect first and second generation relationships and first and third generation relationships?

2. How do mothers feel about their child's divorce, and do these feelings change with time? What are their perceptions regarding the impact of the divorce on their own lives and on the lives of their children?

3. Are changed intergenerational family relationships and/or mothers' attitudes or perceptions regarding the divorce related to the sex of the divorced child?

Additionally, the study provides the opportunity to compare first generation data with previous studies of second generation respondents.

Method

Data in this study were obtained as part of a multidisciplinary study of middle aged and older women (age 50 and over). Women were interviewed twice; once in the summer of 1978 and again in the summer of 1979. Interviews were conducted in the respondents' homes by trained graduate students. The structured interviews included open ended as well as closed ended questions and typically lasted two to three hours.

The original sample of 480 women was obtained by telephoning a random selection of homes in five Madison, Wisconsin census tracts. (The selection of census tracts was based on their high concentration of older people and an attempt to represent the socio-economic make up of the community at large.) If a woman aged 50 or older was identified in the household she was contacted by letter and asked to participate in the study. The 480 participants represent 52% of the eligible women identified in the telephone survey. Four hundred (83%) of the original respondents were interviewed in the second year of this study.

Data for this study on intergenerational effects of divorce were drawn from the second phase of the research. One hundred sixty-nine of the four hundred women (42%) identified at least one relative (son, daughter, sibling, niece, nephew, etc.) who had been divorced. Those reporting divorce in their families were then asked to identify the divorced relative whose divorce had greatest impact on their own lives. Ninety-seven women (24% of the total sample) identified a son or daughter. Of these, seventy-eight had grandchildren by their divorced son or daughter; forty-one of these women had divorced daughters and 37 had divorced sons.

The findings reported here are limited to these 78 grandmothers. The median age of these women was 67 years; age ranged from fifty-two to ninety one. Thirty-seven respondents were married at the time they were interviewed; thirty-one were widowed and ten were divorced or separated. Median family income was approximately $9,000 per year and ranged from $1,000 to $52,000. The respondents averaged three children while their divorced offspring had an average of 2.4 children. The time since the child's divorce ranged from less than one year to 24 years; the average length of time between the divorce and the time of interviewing was eight years.

Results

Effects of Divorce on First & Second Generation Relationships

Behavioral changes were assessed in terms of reported frequency of seeing the divorced son or daughter and former in-law during three time periods: (1) prior to the divorce; (2) year following the divorce; and (3) presently. (Only face to face contact was reported; contact by letter or telephone was not included.) Table 1 summarizes contact with consanguines and affines for the three periods. As might be expected (both in terms of ''common knowledge'' and previous research findings) contact with affines dropped significantly after divorce (p < .001). Although present contact with consanguine kin is not significantly different than prior to the divorce, there was a significant increase in contact with consanguines during the year following divorce (p < .01).

Respondents were asked to rate emotional attachment to consanguines and affines before the divorce and now. Rating was done on a five-point scale with five representing an ''extremely close'' relationship. These results are summarized in Table 2. Respondents were emotionally closer to their affines during the marriage than now (p < .001). Although there was no significant difference in contact with consanguines now and prior to their divorce, respondents reported greater emotional closeness with their offspring now than prior to their divorce (p < .01). It is noted that while there was no difference in contact with affines and consanguines prior to divorce, respondents were notably less emotionally attached to affines during the marriage.

Respondents were asked to provide an overall rating of the extent to which the divorce had affected their relationship with their son or daughter. Seventy six percent (*N* = 59) reported the divorce had not changed this relationship. About 15% (*N* = 12) reported the divorce had changed

Table 1

FREQUENCY OF FIRST & SECOND GENERATION FACE TO FACE CONTACT WITH CONSANGUINES AND AFFINES

Frequency of Contact	Consanguine			Affine		
	Marriage N=77	Year Following Divorce N=76	Now N=75	Marriage N=69	Year Following Divorce N=66	Now N=67
Almost daily	7.8	26.3	14.7	4.3	1.5	1.5
2-3 times per week	14.3	14.5	13.3	13.0	-	-
About once a week	20.8	13.2	18.7	21.7	6.1	7.5
2-3 times a month	9.1	5.3	5.3	10.1	10.6	3.0
About once a month	7.8	9.2	6.7	11.6	4.5	1.5
A few times a year	24.7	19.7	24.0	30.4	13.6	11.9
About once a year	10.4	7.9	9.3	5.8	19.7	10.4
Less than yearly	5.2	3.9	8.0	2.9	43.9	64.2
	100%	100%	100%	100%	100%	100%
Mean[a]	4.636	5.329	4.747	4.594	2.424	1.970
Standard Deviation	2.058	2.294	2.279	1.826	1.772	1.705

[a] Less than yearly = 1; almost daily = 8

Table 2

EMOTIONAL ATTACHMENT TO CONSANGUINES AND AFFINES BEFORE DIVORCE AND NOW

Emotional Closeness	Consanguines		Affines	
	Before Div N=77	Now N=78	Before Div N=74	Now N=72
Not at all close	5.2	3.8	25.7	63.9
Somewhat close	20.8	12.8	31.1	23.6
Quite close	28.6	28.2	24.3	6.9
Very close	40.3	46.2	16.2	5.6
Extremely close	5.2	9.0	2.7	–
	100%	100%	100%	100%
Mean[a]	3.195	3.436	2.392	1.542
Standard Deviation	1.001	.961	1.120	.855

[a] Not at all close = 1; extremely close = 5

the relationship a little or somewhat, while only 9% ($N = 7$) reported quite a bit or a great deal of change. Eighteen of the nineteen who indicated divorce had affected their relationship with their son or daughter provided information about the change. Fifteen women indicated they had more contact, felt closer or reported some other positive change. One woman simply commented that her daughter's life had changed so the relationship now seemed different. Only two respondents indicated a clearly negative change in their relationships with their offspring. One woman noted she was not as close to her son now. The other explained that before the divorce, her daughter "used to come see how she (grandmother) was but now she wants to talk about her own feelings." The two respondents reporting negative changes indicated their relationships with their son and daughter had changed "a little" and "a great deal" respectively. Thus only one of the 78 respondents indicated their child's divorce had produced significant negative change in their relationship.

In summary, respondents reported changes in affine relationships consistent with popular beliefs and previous research findings. Of greater interest were reported changes in relationships with consanguines. Respondents reported significantly more contact with their sons and daughters during the year following divorce than during the marriage and are emotionally closer to their offspring now than during the marriage. Despite this, the overwhelming majority deny that the divorce has changed their relationship with their son or daughter. Fifteen of 19 reported that the divorce produced a positive change in the relationship. Thus it appears that to the extent that divorce effects relationships between first and second generation consanguines, these changes are in the direction of greater emotional closeness between the generations.

Effects of Divorce on First and Third Generation Relationships

Respondents were asked if their contact with their grandchildren had been altered by their child's divorce. (Results are summarized in Table 3.) Forty-two (59.2%) indicated the divorce had not altered contact with grandchildren. Seventeen percent reported increased contact while 24% reported seeing less of their grandchildren following divorce. Roughly half of the respondents who reported decreased contact indicated the decline was substantial. Thus only eight of seventy-one respondents (11.2%) indicated substantial loss in contact with grandchildren following divorce.

Table 3

CHANGE IN CONTACT WITH GRANDCHILDREN AFTER DIVORCE

Type of Change	Daughters N	%	Sons N	%	All N	%
No change	23	63.9	19	54.3	42	59.2
Moderate increase	3	8.3	1	2.9	4	5.6
Substantial increase	4	11.1	4	11.4	8	11.3
Subtotal increase	7	19.4	5	14.3	12	16.9
Moderate decline	3	8.3	6	17.1	9	12.7
Substantial decline	3	8.3	5	14.3	8	11.2
Subtotal decline	6	16.6	11	31.4	17	23.9
	36	100%	35	100%	71	100%

For the group of all grandmothers there were no significant changes in emotional closeness to grandchildren following the divorce. On a five-point scale with 5 indicating an "extremely" close relationship with grandchildren, mean scores were 3.4 and 3.3 respectively for the period prior to divorce and presently.

Respondents were asked whether or not they thought the divorce had changed their relationship with their grandchildren. (See Table 4.) Twenty-one (28%) indicated it had, but only eighteen provided an explanation of the way in which the relationship had changed. Of these, ten reported negative change in their relationship with grandchildren. Three of these indicated negative change with a child of one sex, but not the other.

Respondents were questioned regarding their feelings about recent legislation which granted grandparents visitation rights to their grandchildren as a part of divorce proceedings. The overwhelming majority (89.3%) approved of the legislation. About 7% felt neutral about it, seeing it as neither good nor bad. Only 4% disapproved.

These results indicate that most grandmothers did not see the divorce

Table 4

CHANGE IN RELATIONSHIP WITH GRANDCHILDREN AFTER DIVORCE

Type of Change	Daughters		Sons		All	
	N	%	N	%	N	%
Positive change	4	10.5	4	10.8	8	10.7
Negative change*	3	7.9	7	18.9	10	13.3
Type of change not reported	---	---	3	8.1	3	4.0
Subtotal with change	7	18.4	14	37.8	21	28.0
No change	31	81.6	23	62.2	54	72.0
Total	38	100%	37	100%	75	100%

*Two maternal and one paternal grandmother reported negative change with relationship of child of one sex but not the other.

of their child as having an effect on their relationship with their grand-children. Of those reporting a change in their relationship with grand-children, about half reported a closer relationship. Only about eleven percent reported a significant decline in contact with their grandchild. A similar percentage (13%) identified a negative change in the grandparent-grandchild relationship in response to an open-ended question regarding changes in their relationship with grandchildren. Nearly all of the respondents approved of a court decision granting visitation rights to grandparents in a divorce case.

Respondent's Feelings About Child's Divorce

Respondents were questioned about their feelings toward their child's divorce at the time it occured and at the time they were interviewed. Nine feeling states were identified and women were asked to rate the extent to which they experienced each feeling in regard to their child's divorce. These findings are summarized in Table 5. The strongest feelings at the time of divorce were feelings of unhappiness, sadness, and being upset. On the average mothers tended to be at least somewhat supportive of their child's divorce. Few women felt any guilt over the divorce. Respondents experienced considerable change in their feelings since the divorce. There was a significant (p ≤ .001) decline in the strength of the six of the nine feelings (anger, surprise, unhappiness, being upset, disappointment, and sadness).

Respondents were asked to assess the impact of their child's divorce on their own life; they were also asked to evaluate the impact on the child's life (see Table 6). A similar percentage saw the divorce as having a negative impact on their own lives and on the life of their child (about 24% and 22% respectively). However, only about 3% saw the divorce as having a serious negative impact on their own lives. The majority (61.5%) of the grandmothers saw their child's divorce as having neither a positive nor a negative impact on their own lives; but only 21.7% felt the divorce had no impact (or a neutral impact) on their childen's lives. Most grandmothers (55.1%) saw the divorce as having a positive impact on their child's life. About 12% felt the divorce had a positive impact on their own lives.

Differences between Mothers of Sons and Mothers of Daughters

Several interesting differences emerged between mothers of sons and mothers of daughters. Only one of these differences is consistent with research findings that women are the family "kin keepers." Mothers of sons reported significantly more emotional attachment to their in-law during the marriage than mothers of daughters (i.e., there was greater emotional attachment to female affines than male affines). However, there were no significant sex differences in attachment to the former in-law after divorce.

While divorced daughters see significantly more of their mothers than do divorced sons (p < .05), this does not necessarily support the women as kin keepers theory. Rather it appears to be part of a differing pattern of parental contact for men and women following divorce. This information is summarized in Table 7 and illustrated graphically in Figure 1. Daughters saw somewhat more of their mothers prior to divorce than did sons, but not significantly more. Contact for both sons and daughters increased during the year following divorce and was quite similar for both sexes during this period. The increase for sons is statistically significant, (p < .05) but the p value for daughters slightly exceeds .05. Daughters' present contact with their mothers was virtually the same as during the year following divorce, but sons' contact declined so that it was about the same as prior to divorce. Thus, at present, daughters see significantly

Table 5

MEAN SCORES OF FEELINGS ABOUT DIVORCE

Feeling States	N	After Divorce	Now
Anger*	72	2.15[a]	1.32
		(1.38)[b]	(.95)
Surprise*	70	2.34	1.24
		(1.47)	(.69)
Support	68	2.60	2.76
		(1.50)	(1.46)
Guilt	71	1.15	1.10
		(.65)	(.54)
Unhappiness*	70	3.09	1.83
		(1.46)	(1.39)
Relieved	69	2.25	2.43
		(1.51)	(1.41)
Upset*	69	3.23	1.59
		(1.44)	(1.23)
Disappointed*	67	2.12	1.33
		(1.49)	(.77)
Sad*	69	3.57	2.22
		(1.32)	(1.50)

[a] 1 = Not at all
   2 = Somewhat
   3 = Quite
   4 = Very
   5 = Extremely

[b] Stnadard deviations are in parentheses

*$p < .001$

Table 6

IMPACT OF CHILD'S DIVORCE ON RESPONDENT'S

LIFE AND ON LIFE OF DIVORCED CHILD

	Own Life N=78	Child's Life N=68
Very negative	2.6	7.2
Somewhat negative	21.8	14.5
Neither positive or negative	61.5	21.7
Somewhat positive	7.7	34.8
Very positive	6.4	20.3
	100%	100%
Mean[a]	2.936	3.470
Standard Deviation	.811	1.190

[a] 1 = Very Negative
   5 = Very Positive

more (p < .05) of their mothers than do sons. This was the only time period for which contact differed significantly by sex. There were no sex differences in mothers' emotional attachment to their divorced child either before divorce or now.

There was a trend toward some differences between mothers of sons and mothers of daughters regarding their relationship with grandchildren. (See Tables 3 and 4.) These differences are probably largely explained by the greater likelihood of the divorced woman to have custody of the children (p = .01). Of 72 women reporting the custody disposition of minor grandchilden, 83.8% of mothers of daughters reported their daughter had custody of children while 20% of the sons were reported as having custody.[1] Other custody arrangements (i.e., relative other than parent granted custody, joint or split custody) were reported by ten grandmothers with somewhat more mothers of sons ($N = 7$) reporting those alternate arrangements.

Although the two groups of grandmothers reported similar emotional

---

[1] Father custody exceeds 7% national estimates of fathers with custody.

attachment of their grandchildren prior to divorce, there is some tendency
for mothers of daughters to report more emotional attachment to grandchildren now than do mothers of sons (p = .064). Mothers of daughters
are less likely to report a decline in contact with their grandchildren
following divorce. Of the seventeen who reported seeing less of their
grandchildren, eleven were mothers of sons. Five of eight grandmothers
who reported seeing quite a bit or a good deal less of their grandchildren
were mothers of sons. Mothers of daughters were less likely to report
changes in their overall relationship with their grandchildren (p = .062).
Of the eighteen grandmothers identifying the direction of change in the
relationship eight reported increased contact or other improvements
in the relationship; four of these women were mothers of sons. Seven
mothers of sons (18.9%) and three mothers of daughters (7.9%) reported
negative changes in relationships with grandchildren. Of the mothers of
daughters reporting negative changes in relationships with grandchildren,
one indicated the grandchildren now lived much farther away and another
noted only the relationship with her grandson had suffered. Two mothers

Table 7

FIRST AND SECOND GENERATION CONTACT BY SEX FOR THREE TIME PERIODS

Frequency of Contact[a]	Daughters			Sons		
	Marriage N=40	Year of Divorce N=40	Now N=40	Marriage N=37	Year of Divorce N=36	Now N=36
Almost daily	12.5	22.5	17.9	2.7	30.6	11.1
2-3 times a week	17.5	22.5	20.5	10.8	5.6	5.6
About once a week	20.0	15.0	23.1	21.6	11.1	13.9
2-3 times a month	7.5	2.5	5.1	10.8	8.3	5.6
About once a month	5.0	7.5	2.6	10.8	11.1	11.1
A few times a year	25.0	20.0	20.5	24.3	19.4	27.8
About once a year	7.5	5.0	2.6	13.5	11.1	16.7
Less than yearly	5.0	5.0	7.7	5.4	2.8	8.3
	100%	100%	100%	100%	100%	100%
Mean[a]	4.950	5.450	5.359	4.297	5.194	4.083
Standard Deviation	2.160	2.264	2.230	1.913	2.352	2.170

[a]Less than yearly = 1; almost daily = 8

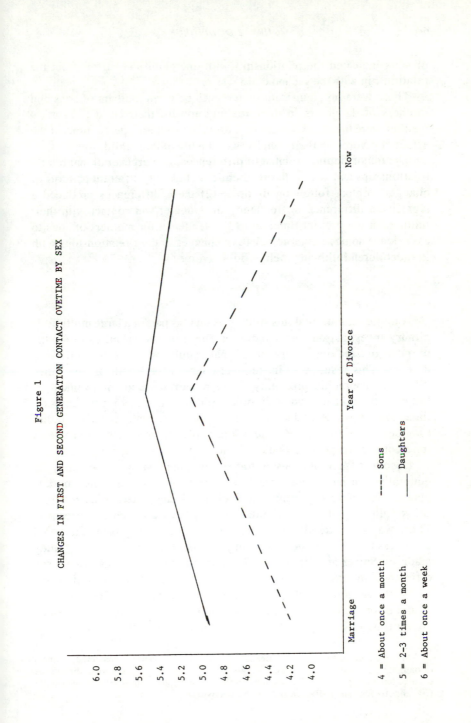

Figure 1

CHANGES IN FIRST AND SECOND GENERATION CONTACT OVETIME BY SEX

4 = About once a month
5 = 2-3 times a month
6 = About once a week

--- Sons

⎯ Daughters

Marriage   Year of Divorce   Now

6.0
5.8
5.6
5.4
5.2
5.0
4.8
4.6
4.4
4.2
4.0

of sons indicated the relationship with one child had suffered but the relationship with the second child was unchanged.

There were no significant differences between mothers of sons and mothers of daughters in their feelings toward their child's divorce.[2] Neither were there differences regarding the women's perceptions of the effect of divorce on their own lives or the life of their child.

The major findings related to differences in intergenerational family relationships and sex of divorced child include: (1) different patterns of changed contact following divorce; (2) these differences produced a significant difference in frequency of daughter/son contact with their mothers at the present time; and (3) a tendency for mothers of sons to experience somewhat more negative changes in their relationships with grandchildren following their child's divorce.

Discussion

A major limitation of this study was that, as part of a large multidisciplinary investigation, the sample was not selected specifically for the purpose of studying intergenerational family relationships following divorce. This resulted in inadequate controls for length of time since divorce, geographic proximity, age, remarriage and involvement of father with child following divorce. Additionally, there was heavy reliance on retrospective data. Given the age of respondents and the rather long periods of time some were asked to recall, the reliability problems inherent in retrospective studies cannot be ignored.

Despite these limitations in study design, the findings of this study are generally consistent with previous studies which questioned middle generation divorced persons about changed intergenerational relationships following divorce. Contact with affines dropped significantly. There was also a trend toward increased contact with greater emotional closeness to consanguines following divorce. However, unlike the study made by Spicer and Hampe (1975) this study found no significant sex differences in contact or emotional closeness to affines following divorce.

While daughters had significantly more contact with their mothers than did sons (consistent with Spicer and Hampe's findings), this difference needs to be explored within the context of differing patterns of

---

[2] When all mothers of divorced sons and daughters ($N = 97$) were considered, mothers of daughters were significantly more supportive than mothers of sons both at the time of divorce and now ($p \leq .05$). For the subsample of grandmothers the p value exceeded .05 (.09 and .07 for time of divorce and now respectively).

changed contact following divorce. It will be recalled that mothers of sons reported greater increase in contact during the year following divorce than did mothers of daughters. However, mothers of sons reported that contact had now returned to predivorce levels, while mothers of daughters indicated contact now was virtually the same as during the year following divorce. We can only speculate about this sex difference in contact patterns following divorce. The differences may be related to the fact that somewhat more sons than daughters have remarried: forty percent of daughters and fifty-four percent of sons were remarried. Although these sex differences are not statistically significant the trend is consistent with the national remarriage statistics. As new spousal and kin relationships are acquired through remarriage there may be less need to maintain the higher level of contact with consanguines. Secondly, since the increase in contact between mothers and sons was reported only for the year following divorce it may suggest that men rely on family support during the immediate postdivorce crisis period but do not continue to use the family as a support system once the initial crisis has passed. However, as custodial parents, women may continue to have greater needs for ongoing support from consanguines. Thirdly, Table 5 suggests there may be a greater tendency for men to return to the parental home following divorce. During the year following divorce, thirty percent of mothers of sons reported daily contact with sons while only six percent reported contact two to three times per week. Although a similar percentage of mothers of daughters reported daily contact a considerably larger percentage (23%) also reported contact several times weekly. Since so few mothers of sons reported contact several times a week, it may be that many of those reporting daily contact actually shared their residence during this period. Men, as noncustodial parents, are less likely to retain possession of their family home and may return temporarily to the parental home.

Some evidence was found of negative changes in grandparent-grandchild relationships following divorce. About ten percent of the sample reported substantial negative change in contact with grandchildren; a similar percentage reported a negative change in their overall relationship with grandchildren. It should be noted, however, that the majority of grandmothers felt their relationship with their grandchildren had not been changed by the divorce, and of those identifying changes in these relationships roughly half reported positive changes.

There was some support for the hypothesis that relationships of paternal grandparents suffer more than those of maternal grandparents.

Even so, only fourteen percent of paternal grandmothers reported a considerable decline in contact with grandchildren following divorce and nineteen percent reported overall negative changes in their relationships with grandchildren. Given popular stereotypes (i.e., divorce leads to family dissolution) and previous research, the importance of our findings may be that relatively few grandmothers saw their relationship with their grandchildren as seriously harmed by their child's divorce.

We have relatively little information about the importance of the grandparent role in the lives of older people. Even if a woman indicates substantial decline in contact with grandchildren, does this necessarily represent a serious negative impact on her own life? In reviewing the available literature on the role of grandparenthood in the lives of older people Wood and Robertson (1976) concluded "there is little indication that most older people find this any more than a symbolic role." In their own research, Wood and Robertson (1978) concurred with Blau (1973) that peer relationships are much more important to older people than are their relationships with their grandchildren or their children. Although this study did not yield information on the importance of the grandparent-grandchild relationship, a large majority of the grandmothers supported the Wisconsin statute providing legal rights to visitation of grandchildren.

Conclusions

The findings of this study suggest that mothers are an important source of support to their divorced children, particularly in the stressful period immediately following divorce. Given the limitations imposed by retrospective data in this study, research conducted with families during the year of crisis is needed to further understand the resources of the extended family as a support system for the divorcing. Information regarding men's support systems is particularly lacking.

Although the majority of grandmothers experienced no major changes in family relationships following divorce it is important not to overlook the twenty percent who reported negative changes in their relationships with grandchildren. Given the current rate of divorce, twenty percent represents a sizeable number of grandmothers who may experience a decline in relationships with grandchildren following divorce. The recently revised Wisconsin divorce statute, providing grandparents the right to petition the court for visiting privileges, addresses the needs of this latter group of grandmothers. However, this provision also appears to have far-reaching implications for policy governing intergenerational family relationships. For example, do grandparents have visitation "rights" only if their children are divorced? What is reasonable visitation for grandparents—weekly, monthly, or holidays and special occasions? Should any grandparent (regardless of their child's marital status) be able to petition the court if dissatisfied with their contact with grandchildren? Is it desirable for courts rather than parents to moderate the grandparent-grandchild relationships? These questions are but a few which may lead to the reexamination of the implications of legally protecting the first and third generation relationships after divorce in the middle generation.

Investigating the effects of divorce and remarriage on intergenerational family relationships is a necessary component to understanding changing patterns of family life. The reorganization of the nuclear family through divorce is a complex process which affects extended kinship obligations and relationships. The family patterns that emerge post-divorce are varied. Some grandparents acquire new relationships, i.e., stepgrandchildren, while others may lose relationships, i.e., an angry custodial mother may prevent visitation of paternal grandparents. Research exploring these changed family patterns across the three generations would provide needed information to families in the transitional process. Additionally, it will lay the necessary groundwork for family policy aimed at strengthening families undergoing change.

REFERENCES

Ahrons, C. R. The binuclear family: two households, one family. *Alternative Lifestyles*, 1979, *2*, (4), 499-515.

Ahrons, C. R. Divorce: a crisis of family transition and change. *Family Relations*, 1980a, *29* (4) 533-540.

Ahrons, C. R. Joint custody arrangements in the postdivorce family. *Journal of Divorce*, Spring, 1980b, *3* (3), 189-205.

Ahrons, C. Redefining the divorced family: A conceptual framework. *Social Work*, 25 Nov. 1980c, 437-441.

Ahrons, C. R. The continuing coparental relationship between divorced spouses. *American Journal of Orthopsychiatry*, 1981, 51 (3), 415-428.

Anspach, D. Kinship and divorce. *Journal of Marriage and the Family*, *38*, May, 1976, 323-330.

Blau, Z. *Old Age in a Changing Society*. New York: New Viewpoints, 1973.

Bohannan, P. Divorce chains, households of remarriage and multiple divorces. In P. Bohannan (ed.) *Divorce and After*. New York: Doubleday and Company.

Furstenburg, F.F., Jr. Recycling the family: perspectives for a neglected family form. *Marriage and Family Review*, 1979, *2* (3), p1, 12-22.

Gongla, P. and Wales, J. Kinship relations after marital separation. Manuscript.

Hetherington, E.M., Cox, M., and Cox, R. Divorced fathers. *The Family Coordinator*, 1976, *25*, 417-428.

Kennedy, P. and Pfeifer, N. *Parents as Intergenerational Mediators: A Conceptual*

Framework and Preliminary Interview Schedule For Studying the Three Generation Family. Unpublished M.S.S.W. thesis, University of Wisconsin, School of Social Work, 1973.

Robertson, J. Interaction in three generation family—parents as mediators: toward a theoretical perspective. *International Journal of Aging and Human Development*, 6 (2), 1975, 103-110.

Shanas, E. *Family Relationships of Older People*. Chicago: Health Information Foundation, 1961.

Spicer, J.W. and Hampe, G.D. Kinship interaction after divorce. *Journal of Marriage and the Family*, *37*, February, 1975, 113-119.

Townsend, P. *The Family Life of Old People*. London: Routledge and Keagan Paul, 1957.

Wallerstein, J.S. and Kelly, J.B. Children and divorce: a review. *Social Work*, 1979, *24* (6), 468-475.

Weiss, R. *Marital Separation*. New York: Basic Books, 1975.

Wisconsin Statutes. Chapter 105, Section 35, 247.245(4), 1977.

Wood, V. and Robertson, J. The significance of grandparenthood. In J. Gubrium (ed.), *Time, Roles, and Self in Old Age*. New York: Human Sciences Press, 1976.

Wood, V. and Robertson, J. Friendship and kinship interaction: differential effect on the morale of the elderly. *Journal of Marriage and the Family*, May, 1978, 367-375.

SUPPORT OF THE PARENT WHEN AN ADULT
SON OR DAUGHTER DIVORCES

Elizabeth S. Johnson
Barbara H. Vinick

ABSTRACT. The impact of a son or daughter's divorce on the older parent has been neglected by researchers and practitioners. Because of the greater needs of the divorcing couple, the impact of divorce on their parents has been largely ignored. Such a divorce may have far reaching implications for the older parent-adult child relationship. Support to the parent primarily from individual friends, other family or clergy may be affected by the view of divorce that these groups hold. Much of the existing literature on divorce focuses almost exclusively on the impact of divorce on the spouses. One could conclude that the divorce of adult sons or daughters is not problemmatic for the parents. We take issue with that conclusion and in the discussion which follows offer evidence and speculation to support our thesis.

In their 1967 book on *Culture and Aging*, Clark and Anderson note that the best potential for good relationships exists between parents and their adult children when both parties are functioning well, when their need to be dependent on each other is minimal. Furthermore they state that the potential for conflict increases when the parents have demands for aid in the form of finances or other support placed on them by their

Elizabeth S. Johnson is a Staff Associate, John Snow Public Health Group, Inc., 210 Lincoln Street, Boston, MA 02111. Barbara H. Vinick is a Research Associate in the Sociology Department at Boston University, Boston, MA 02215. Reprint requests should be directed to the senior author.

child at a time when the parents are beginning to conserve their resources.

Accounts of relations between older parents and their adult children have been given by many researchers (see for example, Brody, 1966; Johnson, 1978; Johnson & Bursk, 1977; Lopata, 1973; Shanas, 1979; Sussman, 1976; Townsend, 1957; Treas, 1977; Troll et al., 1979) and practitioners (see among others, Grollman & Grollman, 1978; Otten & Shelley, 1976; Silverstone & Hyman, 1976). The reports all tend to come to the same conclusion or implication: that despite the problems that exist in some older parent-adult child relationships, the strong bond between parents and their children continues as both grow older. Furthermore, Ethel Shanas (1979) notes that in 1975, the majority (75 percent) of older parents either lived with or lived within a half hour's distance of an adult child and that 77 percent had seen a child during the week prior to their interview.

In another area involving interpersonal relations, that of divorce, there has also been much published: the extent of divorce in the United States (Jacobson, 1959; National Center for Health Statistics, 1977; Norton & Glick, 1979), the social and cultural forces which are related to the phenomenon of divorce (Ackerman, 1963; Bohannon, 1970; Freed & Foster, 1969; Scanzoni, 1979), the effects of divorce on the divorcing couple (Goode, 1956; Gordon, 1976; Hunt, 1966; Weiss, 1975), divorce as a solution to marital discord (Nye & Berardo, 1973) and the effects of divorce on children (Bane, 1979; Glueck & Glueck, 1950; Kalter, 1977; Magrab, 1978; Nye, 1957).

There has been, however, relatively little research or even speculation regarding the effects of divorce on the parents or other extended family members of the divorcing couple. Because of the intense upheaval in the lives of the divorcing spouses, the after shocks in the lives of those outside of the disrupted household have been largely ignored even though network analysis and systems theory suggest that the emotional effects of divorce would not be confined only to the couple and their children.

In view of the important functions served by informal support systems such as the family, the possible turmoil in intergenerational relations which may be initiated by marital breakup seems worthy of study.

Parent and Adult Child Relationships

Relatively little is known about the extent of support offered to the younger divorcing couple by their respective parents or in-laws, although a few researchers have begun to examine the situation from the divorced child's point of view. Anspach (1976) completed a study of contacts of 128 married, divorced, and remarried women with their own and spouse's geographically-available close kindred, the help patterns between the women and kin, and the consequences on these kin contacts when minor children were part of the network. He found that fewer divorced women contact or receive help from their former spouse's kindred than do married women; in fact 80 percent of the divorced and remarried indicated less contact with their spouse's kindred following their divorce.

Roughly the same percent of divorced and remarried women were in touch with close kindred but the divorcees' contact was primarily with their own kin, while the remarried women divided their contacts between their own kin and their new in-laws. Even when the former spouse's kindred were seen by the still divorced women, they were described as least likely to "help." The remarried women and their children became integrated into their new spouse's kin network. Contact with paternal grandparents for children of divorced parents was related to contact with their father.

Using in-depth interviews with 50 recently divorced persons, Spanier and Casto (1979) reported that 84 percent of their interviewees said that their family and friends had been generally supportive of them during the separation process. For those with unsupportive family or friends, the lack of support seemed to increase the interviewee's separation problems especially their emotional difficulties. Those families who were not supportive tended to have strong feelings against divorce in general. One of the female interviewees reported that she had not even told her mother that she was getting divorced, though she saw her frequently, because she felt that it would be too difficult for her mother, "and she did not want to hurt her."

Spicer and Hampe (1975) interviewed 62 divorced men and 42 divorced women regarding their kinship interaction after divorce and found four consistent patterns: (1) interaction with consanguineal kin remains the same as before the divorce or increases, (2) being a woman and/or having custody of children increases or at least maintains interaction with consanguines and also maintains interaction with former spouse's tion with consanguines and also maintains interaction with former spouse's kin, albeit at a lower level than for consanguines, (3) less interaction with spouse's kin almost always occurs, and (4) of all extended kin, the greatest amount of interaction occurs with parents; less interaction occurs as kin distance increases. This pattern also held for the in-law extended family, with parents-in-law receiving the most interaction of all in-law relatives. Overall, Spicer and Hampe found that affection between divorced persons and their blood kin before and after the divorce helped to maintain kinship interaction. On the other hand, the affectional and/or obligational bond with spouses' kin appeared to be weakened or eliminated after divorce.

Margaret Mead noted her belief that many young divorced women with children try to maintain close ties with their own families and even strive to maintain their children's relationships with their father's parents (1970). She wrote (p. 110), "Such attempts [at maintaining relations are] unsanctioned in our present system which permits the connecting link between the grandparents and the grandchildren to drop out completely [and] are often stormy and hazardous." The difficulties may ensue from the in-law grandparents' attempts to protect their son's rights and privileges. Mead felt that these problems might intensify when the daughter-in-law remarried and a real person replaced the absent father in the household.

Parents' Perspectives

Fewer data are available to shed light on how the divorce of a child is perceived by the parents. In a study by the first author, older suburban women were interviewed regarding their social relationships. Those mothers who had experienced the divorce of a child expressed very strong feelings about the event even when it had occurred a number of years earlier. Although the number of women in the sample who had a divorced child was much too small for generalization, it was apparent that the experience had been difficult for all of those whose children had divorced. For some, particularly the mothers whose daughers had not remarried, the bewilderment occasioned by the separaion and divorce was still present.

One such mother was Mrs. Lord whose daughter Claire has been divorced about 10 years and has not remarried. At the time of the divorce Mrs. Lord almost "went to pieces." The marriage seemed so perfect and the couple so in love when they married, that their separation and divorce were incomprehensible. The divorce still appears to be an enigma to her and in recounting her life history she avoided mentioning either of her sons-in-law.

Mrs. Eisen, another interviewee, has a daughter who was divorced and is now remarried. Two children were born during the first marriage, which she described as "tragic." Because her daughter lived in a foreign country during her marriage, Mrs. Eisen rarely saw her but was in constant telephone contact. During this period Mrs. Eisen spent many hours "crying uncontrollably" for her talented daughter who was "destroying herself." After the daughter's ex-husband died in a house fire, her daughter remarried and her second husband adopted both children. She now characterizes the relationship between her daughter and herself as "close and happy."

A third interviewee, Mrs. Lakowitz, appeared to be distraught over her two daughters' "failed" marriages. Divorce in her own family was unheard of. She was particularly upset at the loss of her younger daughter's husband, a dentist, whom she felt was wonderful both to her and her husband. One of her chief concerns was what would happen to her two daughters now that they had no husbands. She both wished and feared that they would take her into their confidence. The fear seemed to stem from her view that she could be of little help to them.

Mrs. Travers also has two daughters, one of whom has been divorced for 9 years. Her daughter is not interested in remarrying, "she has made a life for herself with women." Mrs. Travers and her husband were proud of their daughter Paula's ability to get along as a single person but they worried that she was living too much for her children and would be lost when they left home. They felt that if Paula remarried she would have security and would avoid loneliness. The Travers' other daughter resents the added attention that they pay to Paula even though she does not resent the financial help they provide.

On the basis of the qualitative information just described, a survey was undertaken regarding the divorce of a child. The preliminary analysis confirms that the divorce of a child is indeed a negative life event for the mothers. Mothers of divorced children regard the separation and divorce as "sad," "traumatic," "disastrous." A very small percentage say the event was "good," primarily because the marriage was so "bad." The remarriage of the child appeared to provide some closure to the experience, with greater peace for the mothers as a result.

Because of the negative moralistic tone that society once adopted (and some individuals still hold) with regard to divorce, the parents may feel that they themselves have somehow failed in their upbringing of a child who divorces. Research has in fact focused on the correlation between divorced parents and divorced adult children (Mueller & Pope, 1977). The simplistic, popular equation of divorce with lack of adjustment may cause parents, in retrospect, to feel uneasy about their parenting experience. Parents who took comfort from their "successfully" launched children, may be less comforted and more bewildered in their "post-parental'' years. Other parents may feel anger because they stayed in a bad marriage for the children's sake and now the children are taking the ''easy way out.'' Strangers become ''family'' when a child marries and that familial relationship is strengthened when grandchildren are added. When a child divorces and grandchildren live with the former son or daughter in-law, contact with grandchildren may be greatly reduced. For the majority of older people to whom the grandparent role has been significant (Robertson, 1977), the loss of that relationship may be traumatic. It is also possible for some parents never to see their child's spouse again once the divorce decision has been announced. In spite of the in-law ''jokes'' which abound in our society, it seems likely that the loss of this relationship or what it signifies, is in addition to the loss of the grandchildren, considerable for many parents.

The present generation of older parents appears to be caught between the traditional views of divorce as anathema and the newer concept of divorce as a reasonable if not desirable, solution. The result of this redefinition may be increased anxiety for the parents at a time when concerns about their own aging may be increasing. To further compound their problems, some of the middle aged parents may have parents of their own about whom they are concerned.

Support for Parents of Divorced Children

The parents of a divorcing couple are expected to be supportive of their child and studies have demonstrated that the majority of parents do offer emotional and/or material aid to children in need. Nevertheless, as we have already noted, the divorce of a child may be a heavy burden for the parents as well, especially among members of religious groups that have traditionally censured or forbidden divorce. As mentioned previously, parents may feel that they have somehow ''failed'' or that peers or society in general fault them, at least in part, for their child's unhappy situation. Moreover, loss of valued relationships with son or daughter-in-law and their families and especially loss of contact with grandchildren may make the divorce of a child especially painful. Added to these factors is the vicarious pain which parents may feel when a child is in difficulty or sorrowing or in need. Almost every parent hopes, somewhat unrealistically, that his or her child will avoid all the hurtful experiences that life can offer, even when the child is grown and has flown the parental nest.

This being the case, where do parents of divorcing children turn when they themselves need support? To our knowledge, there are no organized groups in existence at the national level for such parents. There are no therapy or support groups for parents similar to groups for the divorcing couple and even their children of which we are aware although this does not preclude their existence in scattered locations somewhere in this country. A National Organization of Concerned Grandparents, formed a few years ago by neighbors in a Boston suburb to meet with experts and discuss problems associated with children's divorces was short lived. The founder of the organization, which had some national publicity, continues to receive letters from distraught parents asking for advice.

The sources of support which continue to be most utilized are no doubt friends, other family members, and the clergy. Although the major efforts of religious groups concerned with divorce center around the divorcing couple and their children, none of the clergy with whom we spoke informally considered the problems of older parents to be insignificant. Every religious leader of three major religions—Catholic, Protestant, and Jewish—with whom we spoke had had at least some contact with troubled parents of divorcing children. All based their counsel on the specifics of the individual case (Weinglass, Kressel & Deutsch, 1978). Most felt that with the rising number of divorces in the U.S., the problem was not so much one of the "shame" of divorce as it may have been in previous decades, but of guilt on the part of some parents coupled with loss of contact with grandchildren of fear of financial responsibility. Sometimes, in fact, problems appeared when the divorced child and grandchildren moved back to the parental home. Parents of childen raised in Catholic and fundamentalist Protestant homes, in which condemnation of divorce has been traditional, may be particularly hard hit when children divorce. Such parents may not feel that they can rely on the support of friends and family or even their clergy. For example, Catholics who divorce and remarry are excluded from receiving the sacraments of their faith.[*] Groups such as the North American Conference of Separated and Divorced Catholics are spreading the work that divorced and remarried Catholics are not excluded more generally from religious services (NAC SOC, Note 2), but the issue of excommunication remains a thorny one.

---

[*]The alternative to excommunication is to seek a Church "annulment" of the marriage, a process that although simpler than in the past, is difficult for the adults and their parents.

Conclusion

In summary, the feelings of the parents of the divorcing couple have been largely ignored by all groups interested in the phenomenon of divorce. Although their experience with the divorce of their chidren must necessarily remain subordinate to the interests of the principals, the effects on the parents may be potentially detrimental to their life quality: more so because of the lack of recognized support for their relationships with their child, grandchildren, and even their own elderly parents within the context of their child's divorce.

In an era when more people are living longer and when adult children are a major source of at least emotional support for aging parents, earlier life events which have potential for affecting those relationships and hence the support, deserve analysis.

Perhaps the divorce of a child from his/her spouse has little impact on the life quality of the parents. There has been little examination of the experience from the parent's point of view and hopefully that is the case. However, on the basis of preliminary evidence available from a survey of mothers regarding the divorce of their children, and by inference from the related literature on divorce and intergenerational relationships more generally, it is probable that the divorce of a child has some impact. Magrab (1978) notes that for young children divorce may represent loss, failure in interpersonal relationships and a prelude to difficult transitions to new life patterns. It is possible that these factors may exist for older parents of divorced children as well.

REFERENCES

Ackerman, C. Affiliations: structural determinants of differential divorce rates. *American Journal of Sociology*, 1963, *69*, (1), 13-20.

Anspach, D.F. Kinship and divorce. *Journal of Marriage and the Family*, 1976, *38* (May), 323-330.

Bane, M.J. Marital disruption and the lives of children. In G. Levinger & O.C. Moles (Eds.), *Divorce and Separation*. New York: Basic Books, 1979.

Bohannon, P. (Ed.). *Divorce and After*. Garden City, N.Y.: Doubleday, 1970.

Brody, E. The aging family. *Gerontologist*, 1966, *6*, 201-206.

Clark, M., & Anderson, B.G. *Culture and Aging*. Springfield, Il.: Charles C. Thomas, 1967.

Freed, D.J., & Foster, H.H. Divorce American style. *The Annals*, 1969, 383.

Glueck, S., & Glueck, E. *Unraveling Juvenile Delinquency*. Cambridge, MA: Harvard University Press, 1950.

Goode, W.J. *After Divorce*. New York: Free Press, 1956.

Gordon, S. *Lonely in America*. New York: Simon and Schuster, 1976.

Grollman, E.A., & Grollman, S.H. *Caring for Your Aged Parents*. Boston: Beacon Press, 1978.

Hunt, M.M. *The World of the Formerly Married.* New York: McGraw-Hill, 1966.

Jacobson, P. *American Marriage and Divorce.* New York: Rinehart, 1959.

Johnson, E.S. "Good" relationships between older mothers and their daughters: a causal model." *Gerontologist,* 1978, *18* (3), 301-306.

Johnson, Elizabeth S., & Bursk, B.J. Relationships between the elderly and their adult children. *Gerontologist,* 1977, *17* (1), 90-96.

Kalter, N. Children of divorce in an outpatient psychiatric population. *American Journal of Orthopsychiatry,* 1977, *47,* 40-51.

Lopata, H.Z. *Widowhood in an American City.* Cambridge, MA: Schenkman, 1973.

Magrab, P.R. For the sake of the children: A review of the psychological effects of divorce. *Journal of Divorce,* 1978, *1* (Spring), 233-245.

Mead, M. Anomalies in American post divorce relationships. In P. Bohannon (Ed.), *Divorce and After.* Garden City, N.Y.: Doubleday 1970, 97-123.

Mueller, C.W., & Pope, H. Marital instability: A study of its transmission between generations. *Journal of Marriage and the Family,* 1977, *39* (February), 83-93.

National Center for Health Statistics. *Summary Report, Final Divorce Statistics, 1975.* (Monthly Vital Statistics Report, *26* (2), Supplement.) Washington, D.C.: U.S.G.P.O., 1977.

Norton, A.J., & Glick, P.C. Marital Instability in America: Past, Present and Future. In G. Levinger & O.C. Moles (Eds.), *Divorce and Separation.* New York: Basic Books, 1979.

Nye, I.F. Child adjustment in broken and unhappy broken homes. *Marriage and Family Living,* 1957, 19, 356-361.

Nye, I.F. & Berardo, F.M. *The Family: Its Structure and Interaction.* New York: MacMillan, 1973.

Otten, J., & Shelley, F.D. *When Your Parents Grow Old.* New York: Signet, 1976.

Robertson, J.F. Grandmotherhood: A study of role conceptions. *Journal of Marriage and the Family,* 1977, *29,* 165-174.

Scanzoni, J. A historical perspective on husband-wife bargaining power and marital dissolution. In G. Levinger and O.C. Moles (Eds.), *Divorce and Separation.* New York: Basic Books, 1979.

Shanas, E. Social myth as hypothesis: The case of the family relations of old people. *Gerontologist,* 1979, 19 (1), 3-9.

Silverstone, B., & Hyman, H.K. *You and Your Aging Parent.* New York: Pantheon, 1976.

Spanier, G.B., & Casto, R.F. Adjustment to separation and divorce: A qualitative analysis. G. Levinger & O.C. Moles (Eds.), *Separation and Divorce.* New York: Basic Books, 1979.

Spicer, J.W., & Hampe, G.D. Kinship interaction after divorce. *Journal of Marriage and the Family,* 1975, *37* (February), 113-119.

Sussman, M.B. The family life of old people. In E. Shanas & R. Binstock (Eds.), *Handbook of Aging and the Social Sciences.* New York: Van Nostrand, 1976.

Townsend, P. *The Family Life of Old People.* Routledge and Kegan, Paul, London, 1957.

Treas, J. Family support systems for the aged: Some social and demographic considerations. *Gerontologist,* 1977, *17,* 486-491.

Troll, L.E., Miller, S.J., & Atchley, R.C. *Families in Later Life.* Belmont, CA: Wadsworth, 1979.

Weinglass, J., Kressel, K., & Deutsch, M. The role of the clergy in divorce: An exploratory survey. *Journal of Divorce,* 1978, *2,* 57-82.

Weiss, R.S. *Marital Separation.* New York: Basic Books, 1975.

GRANDPARENT VISITATION:
VAGARIES AND VICISSITUDES

Henry H. Foster, Jr.
Doris Jonas Freed

ABSTRACT. Examination is made of the attitude of the law toward the visitation rights of grandparents in divorce and adoption and state statutes which permit an award of visitation when found to be beneficial to the child. The law tends to have more flexible attitudes toward custody claims of grandparents than those for visitation.

Introduction

The visitation rights of grandparents has been a difficult problem for the courts ever since Little Red Riding Hood made her famous trip to her Grandmother's condominium and found Mr. Lupine in bed and Grandma

Henry H. Foster, JD, LLM, is Professor of Law Emeritus of the New York University School of Law, Visiting Professor of Law, New York Law School, Counsel to the New York law firm of Sperry, Weinberg, Waldman, Wels & Rubenstein, a past Chairman of the Family Law Section of the American Bar Association and is a member of the Editorial Board of the *Journal of Divorce*. Doris Jonas Freed, LLB, LLM, JSD, is a member of the Council of the American Bar Association Family Law Section, Chairperson of its Research and Custody Committees, Counsel to the New York law firm of Olvany, Eisner & Donnelly and is a member of the Editorial Board of the *Journal of Divorce*. Professor Foster and Dr. Freed have co-authored many articles and are the co-authors of several books on Family Law.

This is an abbreviated and updated version of an article which appeared in June 23, 27, 29, 1978 *New York Law Journal,* and another version which was published in 23 *St. Louis Law Journal* 643 (1979).

nowhere to be found.[1] Out of sight, out of mind! The hazards of visitation, real and imaginary, constrain the courts to let sleeping wolves lie, and, in the absence of statute, to withhold legal recognition of the claims of grandparents' rights to visitation.

In the background of the conflict between parental and grandparental interests lies the competition between the parental rights theory regarding child custody and visitation and the ''best interests of the child'' or ''least detrimental alternative'' emphasis of many recent cases.[2] The conflict between these two theories as to the premise for an award of child custody ordinarily is more apparent than real and often is merely a matter of semantics,[3] on the issue of visitation the choice between these alternative perspectives may be crucial to the result in a given case. In the absence of statute, and as a common law proposition, courts have been extremely reluctant to interfere with the prerogatives of a fit custodian[4] and to mandate visitation.

This article will explore briefly the common law regarding the visitation rights, if any, of a non-parent and the statutory change which has been effected in some thirty-two states, including New York, that permits an award of visitation in some cases where such would be a benefit rather than a detriment to the child. In this connection it may be important to note that experts on child development are generally agreed about the importance for the child to maintain on-going meaningful relationships that are beneficial.[5]

The Common Law as to Visitation Rights

In reviewing the common law background it is necessary to make a distinction between the situation where a grandparent or other person not having custody seeks to obtain visitation rights and the case where a grandparent or other person has or has had custody from which a parent seeks to reclaim the child.[6] In the former situation, in the absence of statute, it is difficult to secure visitation rights; in the latter situation, where the other person has or had had *de facto* custody, the court has the alternative of either maintaining the existing custodial arrangement and granting visitation rights to the parent, where indicated, or switching custody to the parent, with or without visitation rights to the *de facto* custodian.[7] In other words, even in the absence of statute, many American courts have been loath to disturb a good custodial arrangement at the request of either a parent or non-parent.[8]

The effect of the parental rights doctrine is manifest, especially in the earlier decisions. A fit parent ordinarily will be entitled to visitation if not custody[9] and visitation may serve as a partial vindication of the superior parental claim to the child in cases where the evidence shows that it would be ill-advised to change custody.[10] The efficacy of the parental rights doctrine also is demonstrated where a parent has custody and some other person seeks visitation with the child. As a common law matter, only in exceptional circumstances will visitation be awarded.

It is fair to state that at common law the general rule was that visitation would not be awarded over a parent's or custodian's opposition.[11] However, the general rule is subject to some exceptions, and, in Pennsylvania at least,[12] appears to have been subordinated to concern over the child's best interests. The three major exceptions to the usual common law rule are: (1) where there was an agreement or stipulation as to visitation, as for example, incident to a divorce proceeding;[13] (2) where the child has resided with the person seeking visitation,[14] as for example, where the child's custody was originally awarded to a parent who lived with grandparents and the custodial parent died and the surviving parent seeks a change of custody to him or her; and, finally, (3) where it is demonstrated that the parent seeking custody is "unfit" under the prevailing notions of fitness at the time.[15]

As is true in the case of custody problems generally,[16] the common law decisions about visitation often are noteworthy for their lack of meticulous fact finding and the overuse of presumptions or generalizations that are of doubtful validity. Even though there are early American decisions stressing that the child's best interests are the major concern in custody decisions, (such as that by Mr. Justice Story in *United States v. Green*,[17] decided in 1824) the parental rights doctrine has and continues to dominate common law decisions as to visitation, where a fit parent who has not contracted otherwise seeks to bar such visitation.[18] Most courts have denied visitation even where there has been a long and meaningful association with the petitioner if the custodial parent opposes a grant of visitation,[19] although there are some California and Pennsylvania decisions to the contrary.[20]

The reasons given in *Reiss* and other common law decisions for denying visitation include the following: (1) Ordinarily the parent's obligation to allow the grandparents visitation is a moral and not a legal one;[21] (2) judicial enforcement of a grandparent's visitation rights would divide parental authority thereby hindering it;[22] (3) the best interests of the child are not furthered by forcing the child into the center of the conflict between parent and the grandparents;[23] (4) where there is a conflict between grandparent and parent, the parent alone should be the judge, without having to account to anyone for his motives in denying visitation;[24] and (5) the ties of nature are the only efficacious means of restoring normal family relations and not the coercive measures which follow judicial intervention.[25]

Obviously, the first reason given for withholding visitation begs the question by giving the result as a reason. The issue is whether or not legal recognition should be given to the grandparent's claim to visitation. The second reason given is not a sound reason for an automatic bar to visitation and at most represents a factor to be considered where it is shown that divided authority would place the child in a double bind. The third reason given above is not convincing because the best interests of the child depend upon the overall circumstances and a gratuitous presumption is not warranted.

A review of the common law cases produces a startling conclusion. In many situations, such as where the grandparents have had *de facto* custody, or the parent seeking custody has not functioned as a parent, it may be easier for grandparents to seek or to retain custody than it is for grandparents to obtain visitation rights. The "best interests of the child" doctrine appears to be more operative on the custody issue than it is on the visitation issue. Assemblyman Noah Goldstein of New York is said to have made something of this phenomenon when in seeking an amendment to section seventy-two of the Domestic Relations Law he pointed out that it was ironic that although a New York grandparent could sue for custody, he could not apply for visitation rights.[26] Despite the irony, however, to the extent the courts have recognized the preferred status of a custodial grandparent over one who has not had custody, the result may be justifiable; and efforts at changing the law should be directed at a liberalization of the rules as to visitation under which the nature and character of the association between grandparents and grandchild becomes an important factor to be considered in the exercise of judicial discretion.

Statutes Permitting Grandparents' Visitation

What might be called "grandmother clauses," if we were tempted to pun, have been enacted in some thirty-two states in order to mitigate the severity and uncertainty of the legal status and standing of grandparents at common law to claim visitation privileges. We have found such statutes in Alabama, Arkansas, Arizona, California, Colorado, Connecticut, Delaware, Florida, Georgia, Hawaii, Idaho, Iowa, Kentucky, Louisiana, Michigan, Minnesota, Missouri, Montana, New Jersey, New Mexico, New York, North Carolina, Ohio, Oklahoma, Oregon, Pennsylvania, Texas, Utah, Virginia, Washington, West Virginia, and Wisconsin, although the statutes differ in details and coverage.[26A]

The New York statute is found in sections seventy-two of the Domestic Relations Law and 240.[27] In its original form, a visitation order could be made with reference to grandparents only when the child's parent or parents were dead.[28] Thereafter, in 1974, the provision was amended to cover not only cases where a parent was deceased but other situations as well "in which equity would see fit to intervene."[29] However, only grandparents are mentioned in the statute. In 1976, section 240 of the Domestic Relations Law was also amended to empower the court in a matrimonial action to provide for reasonable visitation to maternal or paternal grandparents of any child of the parties.

Unfortunately, several of the states having such statutes require that one or both parents be deceased for grandparents to be awarded visitation rights. For example, such appears to be true in California (under the original statute), Kentucky, Michigan, New Jersey (until 1973 law which now permits visitation also in cases where parents are divorced or living in different habitats) and Ohio. Arkansas places no limitation, its statute simply providing that in any divorce or custody cases the court may grant visitation rights to grandparents. Connecticut's statute covers parental decease or separation; Louisiana's provides that after divorce or separation, when a parent dies, his or her parents may be awarded visitation; Minnesota's statute covers the situation where the grandchild has resided with the grandparents or they have had considerable personal contact with the child and a parent is deceased or the parents seek a divorce. Texas merely provides that grandparents may be considered for visitation or custody; and Wisconsin that grandparents or great-grandparents may be awarded visitation when it is in the best interests of the child. Oklahoma's unique statute seems to provide that grandparents have visitation rights with their grandchildren unless they are terminated by court order, and that these rights persist even though the child in question is adopted by a stepparent.[30]

In most states the statutes make no reference to the situation where a grandchild is adopted or to the effect of an adoption on the visitation rights of grandparents. In addition to Oklahoma, reference is made to adoption in the California[31] and Minnesota[32] statutes. California now permits visitation rights to be awarded to a grandparent where the adoption is by a stepparent or other grandparent, but not otherwise, and Minnesota's statute is to the same effect. Since the problem regarding the effect of an adoption upon the visitation rights of grandparents arises with some frequency, and the cases are in conflict,[33] it is wise to cover the matter by an express statutory provision, and the distinction made between an adoption by a stepparent or grandparent and that by a stranger has considerable merit.[34] We understand that the Louisiana legislature currently is considering a bill which would permit grandparent visitation after adoption.[35]

The state statutes also differ on whether or not relatives other than grandparents may seek and obtain visitation rights. California permits visitation to be accorded "anyone interested in the welfare of the child."[36] Connecticut permits visitation to be awarded to any "third party including but not limited to grandparents,"[37] and Hawaii also permits visitation to be awarded to "any other person having an interest in the welfare of the child."[38] Ohio provides that relatives may be granted visitation.[39]

As in New York, many of these statutes are qualified so that it must be found that visitation is in accordance with the best interests of the child. Minnesota directs the court to consider the amount of personal contact between the grandparent and the child,[40] and Idaho requires a substantial relationship with the child.[41] Although it may be superfluous to write such a requirement into the statute, such provisions have the advantage of emphasizing the important factor of the psychological relationship between the child and the party seeking visitation.

A sound argument may be made that any person or relative, in addition to a grandparent, should have standing to seek visitation rights where he or she has maintained a substantial relationship with the child.[42] It may be in the best interests of the child to grant an aunt,[43] or uncle,[44] or even a non-relative visitation. Further, the grant of visitation should not be restricted necessarily to cases where there has been a parental divorce or one or both parents have died. As expressed in the Idaho and Minnesota statutes, the crucial question should be the child's welfare. Assuming the existence of a meaningful and beneficial relationship with a relative or a third person, it may be more important to the child to preserve that relationship than it would be for the custodian to have an absolute veto power over visitation.

In the approximately twenty-one states, which do not have statutory provisions granting discretion to award visitation rights to non-parents, legislative consideration should be given not only to the policy basis for mitigating the common law but also to an extension of visitation rights to relatives and non-relatives who have stood *in loco parentis* or have a substantial interest in the welfare of the particular child.

Several interesting issues have emerged as a result of the statutory construction and judicial interpretation of visitation provisions. California in particular has decided a series of cases which highlight two emergent issues, namely the effect of an adoption of the child on the statutory visitation privilege, and the impact of animosity or hostility between the custodian and the party seeking visitation on discretionary awards of visitation.

Odell v. Lutz,[45] decided in 1947 before there were any statutory visitation privileges, followed earlier California cases[46] and on a common law basis denied a maternal grandmother visitation with her grandchild who had been adopted by the father's second wife. In reaching that decision the court said that

> [T]he state may not constitutionally interfere with the natural liberty of parents to direct the upbringing of their children . . . The supremacy of the father and mother in their own home in regard to the control of their children is generally recognized . . . There is nothing in the record which would indicate that the association of the plaintiff and her grandchild would be anything other than beneficial to the child. However, the court does not have the power to compel the parents to allow the grandmother the right of visitation merely because the relationship is that of grandparent.[47]

The common law rules regarding visitation by grandparents were altered by the enactment of section 197.5 of the Civil Code which permitted visitation orders in favor of grandparents in cases where the grandparents' child was deceased. Under this provision it is necessary to qualify as the parent of a deceased child in order to seek visitation rights as a grandparent[48] and statutory procedure must be adhered to.[49] The California Family Law Act, which became effective in 1970, in section 4601 of the Civil Code expands upon visitation and provides:

> Reasonable visitation rights shall be awarded to a parent unless it is shown that such visitation would be detrimental to the best interests of the child. In the discretion of the court reasonable visitation rights may be granted to any other person having an interest in the welfare of the child.

In a series of cases the California courts have considered the effect of adoptions of the child on the visitation rights of grandparents. In *Roquemore v. Roquemore*,[50] while an action for visitation was pending, and after temporary visitation rights had been awarded to the paternal grandparents, the mother's second husband adopted her son. Her first husband, the father of the child in question, was deceased, and his widow remarried. The mother and adoptive father moved to dismiss the petition for visitation brought by the paternal grandparents, and the motion was granted by the trial court. The appellate court reversed, holding that the adoption statute did not preclude an award of visitation rights under the California statutes.

In *Reeves v. Bailey*,[51] the maternal grandparents, without notice to the paternal grandparents, who previously had been awarded visitation rights, adopted the child, allegedly solely for the purpose of cutting off such visitation. Upon appeal there was a reversal of the trial court and it was held that: (1) the paternal grandparents might attack the adoption on the basis of fraud, and (2) that their court-ordered visitation rights were not automatically terminated by the adoption decree when the adoption did not work any major change in the child's living arrangements. The court declared that whether visitation was no longer in the child's best interests or would unduly hinder the adoptive relationship was a matter to be established in a proper proceeding in which all interested parties might participate. *Adoption of Berman*[52] was distinguished on the basis that it involved a denial of visitation rights in a situation where visitation would not have been in the child's best interests. In passing, the California court referred to two New York decisions, citing with approval *Scranton v. Hutter*,[53] and rejecting the rationale of *People v. Rado*.[54]

Maternal grandparents, however, were found to be too litigious and lost in *Adoption of Berman*.[55] There, after the death of their daughter who was the mother of the children in question, the maternal grandparents were granted temporary guardianship of the children. However, when the father remarried, the temporary guardianship was terminated, although the maternal grandparents were granted reasonable visitation rights. A series of court proceedings followed and their visitation rights were reduced and finally complete discretion was given to the father and his second wife regarding terms of visitation. While the visitation proceedings were pending, the second wife adopted the children in another county, no notice being given to the maternal grandparents. The court refused: (1) to set aside the adoption on the ground of fraud, and (2) decided that court-ordered visitation would not be in the best interests of the children in light of the prior hostilities engendered by all of the litigation between the parties.

In addition to the standing accorded grandparents by the California statutes, an agreement or stipulation regarding visitation rights may also give rise to a claim for visitation if visitation is in the best interests of the children. *Benner v. Benner,*[56] reached such result before the enactment of the California statutes, and *Bookstein v. Bookstein,*[57] so held after California's visitation statutes had been enacted. Of course, the court is not bound by the agreement or stipulation where it is shown that visitation would not be in the child's best interests.

New Jersey and Ohio agree with California that a stepparent adoption does not terminate the visitation rights of grandparents. In *Mimkon v. Ford,*[58] the New Jersey court read the adoption and visitation statutes as being *in pari materia* and awarded visitation rights to the maternal grandparents despite an adoption of the child by its stepmother who had married the father after the mother's death. As the California court had done in *Roquemore v. Roquemore,* the New Jersey court made a distinction between an adoption by a relative, such as a stepparent, and an adoption by a stranger. *Graziano v. Davis,*[59] an Ohio decision, discussed the conflict in authorities and held that a stepparent adoption was merely a factor to be considered by the court in the exercise of its discretion to grant or to withhold visitation rights when there had been an adoption. The court rejected cases from Kansas,[60] Louisiana,[61] Texas,[62] and New York,[63] which had held to the contrary.

Unfortunately, judicial analysis of the visitation rights of grandparents, especially where the child in question has been adopted, has been complicated and confused by the assertion that the statutory visitation right of the grandparent is derivative and not an independent right or privilege of grandparents qua grandparents. Although there are decisions that describe the visitation rights of grandparents as "derivative" and which purport to find a basis for that conclusion in statutory language,[64] the better reasoned cases hold the contrary. Thus, *Bennett v. Bennett*[65] concluded that there was nothing in the New Jersey statute which asserts that a grandparent's visitation rights are derivative. In that case, the parties had been divorced in 1974 and custody had been placed with the mother. In 1976 the father sought modificaton but the action was settled by agreement to place custody with the maternal grandparents, with liberal visitation rights to the father as long as visitation took place in the home of the paternal grandparents. Thereafter the father moved to California, failed to exercise his visitation rights, and his mother sought to see the child but was refused access. In reversing the denial of visitation to the paternal grandmother the appellate court directed the trial court to inquire into the possible advantages and disadvantages which might flow from a grant of visitation rights and to set the terms of visitation.

On the other hand, in a questionable decision,[66] New Jersey has held that it would seldom, if ever, be in the best interests of a child to grant visitation to the grandparents when their child, the parent, already had such rights. Since the New Jersey statute specifically provides that a grandparent may be awarded visitation where either or both parents "is or are deceased, or divorced or living separate and apart in different habitats,"[67] it is clear that the visitation rights of the divorced son should not bar additional visitation rights for the paternal grandparents in their own right if circumstances favor the latter. Of course, if the accumulation of visitation rights threatens the legitimate interests of the custodial parent,[68] or is merely a ploy to get additional visitation for their son, the welfare of the child in question may require a denial of further visitation rights to the grandparents. However, the court said that "visitation by grandparents should be derivative" and ignored the statutory language which obviously grants grandparents an independent right to seek visitation. Rather than announcing broad policy or a generalized rule which conflicts with the statute, we feel that the court should have explored the facts and circumstances of the particular case in order to determine whether or not *in fact* the visitation sought was not in the best interests of the child or impaired substantial interests of the custodial parent. Otherwise, in effect, the animosity of the custodial parent may be sufficient to preclude the visitation contemplated by the New Jersey statute.

Other than the problem of reconciling visitation rights or statutes with the law and policy regarding adoptions, the most controversial issue in visitation cases has been what weight, if any, should a court give to the existence of animosity between the parties. As we have seen, the common law regarded the opposition of the custodian as sufficient reason for denying visitation.[69] Where there is statutory recognition of visitation rights the mere existence of animosity alone usually has been regarded as an insufficient reason for withholding them. Perhaps Pennsylvania in *Williams v. Miller*,[71] reached a sensible result, even though there was no visitation statute, when the case was remanded in order for the trial court to determine the basis for any alleged animosity. The trial court in effect also was directed to retain continuing jurisidiction in order to determine what effect, if any, visitation had upon the child's welfare.

An earlier Pennsylvania decision, *Commonwealth ex rel. Goodman v. Dratch*,[72] also held that the existence of animosity between the parties was no bar to an award of visitation rights. The child had lived with his maternal grandparents for nearly a year following the death of his mother until custody was awarded to the father. In response to a showing of friction between the parties and the testimony of a psychologist that visitation with the grandparents would be detrimental to the child's health, the court said "We consider that it would be almost inhuman to completely isolate the child from his grandparents . . . Unless there be some compelling reason, we do not believe that a grandchild should be denied visitation to his grandparents."[73] However, in *Commonwealth ex rel. McDonald v. Smith*,[74] visitation was denied because of the friction between the parties.

Decisions from Georgia[75] and Maryland[76] agree that animosity in and of itself is no bar to an award of visitation rights. In California, family friction in the case of *In re Adoption of Berman*[77] led to a severe restriction of visitation rights, but in *Benner v. Benner*[78] animosity was offset by the fact that the grandparents had raised the child in question for three years.

It is difficult to see why statutory visitation privileges should rest on a basis different from visitation rights generally, such as that by a divorced parent. The existence of animosity or hostility between the divorced parties, in and of itself, is not a ground for withholding visitation. Although there is an esoteric but well-known argument that custodial parents should have a veto power over any and all visitation,[79] there is scant if any legal authority to back up the argument, and in fact, it has been rejected.[80]

At most, animosity may be a matter which invites exploration by the court in order to determine its factual basis, or a factor to be considered in awarding and setting the terms of visitation. Otherwise, as has been pointed out,[81] the custodian may lift himself by his bootstraps by creating friction which he then points to as a reason for denying custody. Moreover, the approach should not be in terms of rewarding or punishing feuding parties, rather the concern should be with the child's best interests. Especially where there has been a meaningful association between the child and the party seeking visitation, the blame for existing hostilities ordinarily is irrelevant unless it has some direct bearing on the child's welfare. Obviously, grandparents may be good grandparents and yet for one reason or another have bad relations with a son or daughter-in-law.

The matter of the child's preference regarding visitation has been accorded the same weight as in custody cases generally. In other words, a stated preference of an older child is a matter to be considered in an exercise of discretion by the court but the child's wishes are not determinative. In *Commonwealth ex rel. Flannery v. Sharp*,[82] the Pennsylvania court gave the child's opposition to visitation as a reason for denying it. The child had said that she did not want to visit the grandparents because "they fight my mother." The Ohio decision in *In re Griffiths*[83] likewise denied visitation because the child disliked the grandparents. The difficulty with these cases is that the child may have been "brainwashed" or may be parroting what the custodial parent told him.

Where there are visitation statutes, a positive desire on the part of the child for visitation should carry great weight, but a negative attitude on part of the child may require further exploration. *Lucchesi v. Lucchesi*,[84] an Illinois decision, approached visitation in terms of the right of the children to know and associate with grandparents and honored the stated preference of the children. In *Ehrlich v. Ressner*,[85] however, the New York Supreme Court, Second Department, held that the trial court had placed undue emphasis upon the grandchildren's opposition to court-ordered visitation.

The effect of visitation upon the health of the child is another important factor in visitation cases as well as in custody cases generally. Where it is shown that visitation would have an adverse effect on the child's health, generally it will be denied.[86] The other side of the coin is shown by *Benner v. Benner*,[87] a California decision, where the court concluded that a termination of contact with grandparents, who had stood *in loco parentis* with the child, probably would have an adverse effect upon the child's health and welfare.

We have enumerated above some of the major factors that courts have regarded as relevant in an exercise of the court's discretion in determining visitation privileges. One factor, of doubtful relevance, is a distinction between natural grandparents and grandparents by adoption.[88] In *Commonwealth ex rel. Dogole v. Cherry*,[89] a mother who had adopted the child died, and her mother, the maternal grandmother, sought visitation rights with the child who remained in the father's custody. Visitation was denied, apparently because the child was not of the same bloodline. This quaint application of the old shibboleth that blood is thicker than water was unwarranted and totally disregards the fact that meaningful relationships do not depend upon blood relationships, as the institution of marriage itself purports to recognize.

Custody Awards to Grandparents

As distinguished from visitation orders secured by grandparents or others pursuant to common law or statute, a related but distinct problem arises where the grandparents of a third person seek child custody rather than visitation. In most cases the controversy has been between a grandparent and a parent, and often the issue is an ancillary one in divorce or dissolution proceedings. Since such custody controversies are the subjects of exhaustive notes and annotations,[90] only a sampling of the cases is necessary.

It is in custody litigation that the competition between the parental rights and child's best interests doctrines have had their most spectacular exposure. Courts which approach custodial decisions with a premise that parents have a proprietary interest in their children ordinarily require a showing of parental unfitness before serious consideration is given to placement of the child elsewhere.[91] When the perspective of the child's best interests is adopted, a non-parent who had had *de facto* custody or who has stood *in loco parentis*, may become the odds on favorite to win custody. Neither premise, however, purports to be absolute, and the use of presumptions may dilute or reinforce whichever doctrine is adhered to.[92]

As has been pointed out elsewhere[93] even the early American decisions usually avoided doctrinaire applications of doctrines and none other than Mr. Justice Story in 1824 stressed the welfare of the child as the chief consideration in determinations of custody.[94] The claims of parents to child custody usually have been conditioned upon a requirement of parental fitness, although there are a few English and nineteenth century American decisions that seem to speak in terms of parental absolutes.[95]

With reference to grandparents in particular, perhaps it is safe to generalize that a grandparent who has stood *in loco parentis* usually will prevail in a custody case over a parent who has been unconcerned and has never assumed the proper care of the child.[96] So too where there is a demonstration of parental unfitness, such as moral delinquency,[97] criminality,[98] brutality,[99] or addiction to drugs or alcohol.[100] Insanity or serious mental illness also may establish parental "unfitness," without regard to fault.[101] Prior abandonment of the child, or a relinquishment or disavowal of parental responsibilities,[102] also may be subsumed under the rubric of parental unfitness. In *Bennett v. Jeffreys*,[103] New York added an amorphous category of other exceptional or extraordinary circumstances, including the situation where the mother let a surrogate care for the child for a number of years, thereby establishing a psychological parent-child relationship.

The more recent cases involving child custody indicate that even where a state has a tradition of adherence to the parental rights theory, an expansion of the concept of parental "unfitness" may lead to the same result as a commitment to the child's best interests theory.[104] However, the result is less certain, and where the child's welfare is the focal point, courts are most apt to give great weight to psychological parent-child relationships or meaningful prior associations with the child.[105] Of course, there is a danger that courts may be overcome by an unconscious bias and abandon common sense under either approach.

In a relatively recent Georgia case,[106] the lifestyles of the parents led to a custody award to grandparents, apparently on the assumption that the grandparents would not compound their previous failure (from the court's point of view) in the rearing of their own child. The parents were regarded as "hippies" by the court, since they smoked pot, adopted a unisex style, and lived in a commune. It was pointed out by the court, however, that both parents had been National Merit Scholars and had graduated from Harvard University. The latter accomplishment may have been the clincher. The well-known decision of the Iowa court in *Painter v. Bannister*,[107] is another example of judicial prejudice regarding lifestyle. The point is that under the "best interests test" there is a special danger that the test or doctrine may be misapplied by self-righteous courts, or middle class case workers,[108] so as to confuse bias with welfare. The special danger of the parental rights approach is that a psychological parent-child relationship may be ignored. Both dangers may be mitigated or avoided by meticulous fact finding and a commitment to objectivity.[109]

As previously discussed, one of the interesting phenomena of custody cases is that there may be a tempting compromise or way out of difficult situations. In denying a parent legal or physical custody, the court may give him the sop of visitation rights, or experimentally, it may award temporary custody to a non-parent and provide for increasing parental visitation and eventual custody.[110] Unless closely supervised, the difficulty here is that the child may be caught in a double bind, as sometimes where joint custody is awarded, and he may become the victim of a judicial compromise of conflicting rights.

An award of custody also may be made as a compromise where a grandparent seeks to adopt and in lieu of adoption is given legal custody.[111]

A different but somewhat similar problem may occur where a natural mother is willing to place her child for adoption on the condition that she retain visitation rights with the child. In the past, agencies have summarily brushed aside such conditional relinquishments for adoption, but with the short supply of readily adoptable children, and the current emphasis on ''roots,'' a reconsideration of policy may be in order.[112] If adoptive parents are willing to accept visitation by the natural mother, and she is a ''fit'' person, there is much to be said for such an arrangement.

Since a few years ago—at least ten—it was reported that the average American woman is a grandmother by age 47—and today the age may be even lower—it is not surprising that great-grandparents should seek custody. In *Cox v. Mills*,[113] the Georgia court held for the mother rather than the great-grandparents of a six-year-old child. Other cases, however, have awarded custody to grandparents where circumstances warranted it.[114]

As previously indicated, there may be a fusion of the parental rights doctrine and the best interests of the child test in custody cases. A substantial annotation of the cases concludes that:

> Clearly the most important single factor which determines whether the welfare of the child is better served by awarding its custody to the father or to the grandparents is the relative fitness of the parties to care for the child. In determining the fitness of the parties the courts have considered a variety of circumstances, but have stressed particularly the moral character and emotional stability of the claimants. If the parent has made an agreement with another person, surrendering to him the custody of the child, such agreement may have weight as showing the unfitness of the parent and stopping him from seeking to repudiate the fair and beneficial agreement; but it will not be enforced as a binding agreement unless it is for the benefit of the child. In addition to the relative fitness of the parties, the courts also have been influenced by various factors which relate primarily to the child, such as his age and sex, his health, and his personal preference.[115]

As previously pointed out with regard to awards of visitation to non-parents, there is no substantive due process objection to a warranted award of custody to a non-parent. Procedural due process, of course, applies to custody proceedings,[116] so that parents are entitled to notice and an opportunity to be heard.[117] Moreover, there is a potential due process issue if a fit parent, without cause, is arbitrarily deprived of the custody of his child;[118] and there may even be an equal protection issue if there is an arbitrary classification of parents subject to termination of their parental rights.[119] It may be assumed that a finding of parental unfitness is not constitutionally limited to a case of moral delinquency and that an impaired physical or mental capacity to function as a parent, the presence of a contagious disease, or other circumstances that make custody with him hazardous to the child, will suffice to support a finding of "unfitness." *Prince v. Massachusetts*[120] seems to support this analysis.

It bears repetition to remark that, curiously, the courts in custody cases seem to have adopted a more flexible attitude towards the custody claims of grandparents than in cases where a grandparent merely asserts rights of visitation. In part this may be due to the common law pronouncement that grandparents had no visitation rights over parental opposition, and usually, Pennsylvania to the contrary notwithstanding, statutes have been necessary to provide legal status to grandparents seeking visitation. In addition, the issue of visitation usually has arisen after custody already has been established or determined, so that it is viewed as a threat to custodial prerogatives. The timing and the situation is different when a parent, for example in a divorce proceeding, is faced with an initial determination regarding placement of the child. There, the door is open wider for a determination in accordance with the child's best interests and the court has the satisfaction of knowing that an award which later may turn out to be a mistake may be corrected in subsequent modification proceedings.

Conclusion

Although only thirty-two states have statutory provisions permitting an award of visitation to grandparents, or other concerned relatives or friends of the child, there currently is greater judicial consciousness of the psychological theory of the importance of existing associations and intergenerational contacts. As we have seen, Pennsylvania, in the absence of statute, has adopted the common law so as to accord visitation rights to grandparents. If the best interests of the child is a meaningful concept, and the focal point in visitation and custody cases, it is clear that it is a sound policy to nurture rather than to cut-off his close relationships.

Even though the parental rights premise is dying a slow death we need not mourn. The law of *potestas* has no validity in contemporary America but we should be careful that we do not adopt a similar approach in determining the visitation rights of grandparents. Properly, the recognition of such rights should be entrusted to the sound discretion of the court. It is not the grandparents' proprietary interest in the grandchild which justifies an award of visitation or custody; it is the need of the grandchild to know and to have an association with concerned grandparents. The pleasures grandparents may derive from that association are merely a bonus, albeit a very precious one.

With reference to the two major issues in the visitation cases, that is, the effect of the child's adoption upon visitation rights, and the weight to be given the existence of animosity between the parties, we conclude that both issues should be approached from the perspective of the child's best interests. Surely stepparent adoption or adoption of the child by other relatives does not require insulation of the child from contact with grandparents or other meaningful associations and it is only in the case of non-relative adoption where an argument may be made that adoption policies demand that visitation be denied. On the issue of animosity and its role in visitation cases, *Lo Presti v. Lo Presti*[121] is correct in concluding that there is no convincing reason why the existence of a state of animosity should have any more effect when grandparents seek visitation than it does where visitation is awarded to the other parent. In either event, it is a circumstance to be considered, but the child's welfare, including his right to maintain meaningful associations, should be the controlling consideration.

FOOTNOTES

1. If 'Lil red had been erudite and had studied her Latin, she would have grabbed hold of Mr. Lupine and cried *aribus teneo lupum*!

2. The "best interests of the child" terminology persists despite Goldstein, Freud and Solnit's, Beyond the Best Interests of the Child (1973), chapter 4, where it is urged that courts adopt "the least detrimental alternative" formula.

3. See Foster and Freed, Child Custody, 39 N.Y.U.L. Rev. 423, 615 (1965).

4. See Note, Visitation Rights of Grandparents Over the Objection of a Parent: The Best Interests of the Child, 15 J. Fam. Law 51 (1976-77); Note, Statutory Visitation Rights of Grandparents'' One step Closer to the Best Interests of the Child, 26 Cath. Univ. L. Rev. 387 (1977); and Gault, Statutory Grandchild Visitation, 5 St. Mary's L.J. 474 (1973).

5. See Goldstein, Freud and Solnit, Beyond the Best Interests of the Child, Chapter 3; Watson, The Children of Armageddon: Problems of Custody Following Divorce, 21 Syracuse L. Rev. 55 (1969); Wallerstein and Kelly, The Effects of Parental Divorce: The Adolescent Experience, in The Child in His Family: Children at Psychiatric Risk, vol. 3 (ed. by Anthony and Koupernik, 1974).

6. See Note, Visitation Rights of a Grandparent Over the Objection of a Parent: The Best Interests of the Child, 15 J. Fam. Law 51, 64 (1976-77); Annot., Visitation Rights of Persons Other Than Natural or Adoptive Parents, 98 A.L.R.2d 325.

7. For example, see Benner v. Benner, 248 P.2d 425 (Cal. App. 1952), and Commonwealth ex rel. Goodman v. Dratch, 192 Pa. Super. 1, 159 A.2d 70 (1960).

8. "Where a grandparent has previously had the custody of the child for so long a period as to stand *in loco parentis*, the courts recognize that a sudden and complete termination of contact between them is likely to cause adverse effects upon the child." Note, Grandparent Visitation, 15 J. Fam. Law 51, 63 (1976-77).

9. Id. However, where both parents are unfit, custody may be awarded to grandparents. See Kees v. Fallen, 207 So. 2d 92 (Miss. 1968); In re Craigo, 266 N.E. 92, 145 S.E.2d 376 (1965); and State ex rel. Obrecht v. Obrecht, 256 S.W.2d 955 (Tex. Civ. App. 1953). Custody will be denied an unfit parent. See Jackson V. Fitzgerald, 185 A.2d 724 (D.C. 1962); Lee v. Kepler, 197 So. 2d 570 (Fla. App. 1967); Kay v. Kay, 51 Ohio Op. 434, 112 N.E.2d 562 (1953) (custodial parents not alleged to be unfit entitled to determine visitation if any); People ex rel. Schachter v. Kahn, 241 App. Div. 686, 269 N.Y.S. 173 (2d Dept. 1934) (grandparents habeas corpus petition dismissed for failure to allege parental unfitness); but compare Chodzko v. Chodzko, 35 Ill. App. 3d 357, 342 N.E.2d 122 (1975) (where maternal grandmother was permitted to intervene in custody proceedings to secure visitation rights without alleging parental unfitness).

10. _____ U.S. _____, 98 S. Ct. 549 (1978).

11. Note, Grandparent Visitation, 15 J. Fam. Law 51, 55 (1976-77). Among the most frequently cited common law decisions are the following: Veazy v. Stewart, 472 S.W.2d 102 (Ark. 1971); Odell v. Lutz, 177 P.2d 628 (Cal. App. 1947); Jackson v. Fitzgerald, 185 A.2d 724 (D.C. Mun. Ct. App. 1962); Succession of Reiss, 46 La. Ann 347, 15 So. 151 (1894); In re Matter of the Adoption of a Child by M, 140 N.J. Super. 91, 355 A.2d 211 (1976); Noll v. Noll, 98 N.Y.S.2d 938 (1950); Kay v. Kay, 112 N.E.2d 562 (Ohio C.P. 1953); Schriver v. Schriver, 7 Ohio App. 2d 169, 219 N.E. 2d 3ll (1966); Commonwealth ex rel. McDonald v. Smith, 85 A.2d 686 (Pa. Super. 1952); Commonwealth ex rel. Flannery v. Sharp 30 A.2d 810 (Pa. Super. 1943); Smith v. Painter, 408 S.W.2d 785 (Tex, Civ. App. 1966), writ of error refused, 412 S.W.2d 28 (Tex. Sup. Ct. 1967); and Green v. Green, 485 S.W.2d 941 (Tex. Civ. App. 1972). For a critique of statutory change in Texas, see Gault, Statutory Grandchild Visitation, 5 St. Mary's L.J. 474 (1973).

12. See Williams v. Miller, 4 F.L.R. 2397 (Pa. Super. 1978) (April 13, 1978). See also Mirto v. Bodine, 29 Conn. Supp. 510, 294 A.2d 336 (1972), where it was held grandparents might seek visitation in an independent action and were entitled to a hearing on the best interests of the child and their intervention was not limited to divorce proceedings. Evans v. Lane, 8 Ga. App. 826, 70 S.E.2d 603 (1911), awarded visitation to the maternal grandmother, without statutory aid, where her daughter had died shortly after childbirth, despite the enmity existing between her and her son-in-law. These and other cases may be sufficient to comprise a minority common law position.

13. See A.L.R.2d 325, 328-29 (1964); Benner v. Benner, 248 P.2d 425 (Cal. App. 1952). Compare People ex rel. Marks v. Grenier, 249 App. Div. 564, 293, N.Y.S.2d 364 (1st Dept.), affirmed, 274 N.Y. 613, 10 N.E.2d 577 (1937); and Woods v. Parkenson, 430 P.2d 467 (Colo. 1967). See also Note, 15 J. Fam. Law 51, at 68, and Bookstein v. Bookstein, 7 C.A.3d 219, 86 Cal. Rptr. 495 (1970); Scott v. Scott, 154 Ga. 659, 115 S.E. 2 (1922); and Minge v. Minge, 226 Ark. 262, 289 S.W.2d 189 (1956) where the father failed to pay support, it was not an abuse of discretion to award grandparents visitation two Sundays a month.

14. See Annot., 98 A.L.R.2d 325, 328-29 (1964), and Benner v. Benner, 248 P.2d 425 (Cal. App. 1952). It has been held that grandparents have a limited right to intervene in divorce proceedings in order to seek custody or visitation. Id.

15. See cases cited op. cit. supra note 9.

16. See Foster and Freed, Life With father: 1978, 11 Fam. Law Q. 321 (1978).

17. 26 F. Cas., 30 (D.R.I. 1824) No. 15,256.

18. See cases cited op. cit. supra note 11, and also Browning v. Tarwater, 215 Kan. 501, 524 P.2d 1135 (1974).

19. See the citation of authorities in Mimkon v. Ford, 66 N.J. 426, 332 A.2d 199 at 201 (1975).

20. See cases cited op. cit. supra note 12.

21. See Gault, Statutory Grandchild Visitation, 5 St. Mary's L.J. 474, 480-81 (1973); Succession of Reiss, 46 La. Ann. 347, 15 So. 151 (1894); and Smith v. Painter, 408 S.W.2d 785 (Tex. Civ. App. 1966), writ of error refused, 412 S.W.2d 28 (Tex. Sup. Ct. 1967).

22. See Odell v. Lutz, 177 P.2d 628 (Cal. App. 1947); and Jackson v. Fitzgerald, 185 A.2d 724 (D.C. Mun. Ct. App. 1962).

23. For example, see Noll v. Noll, 98 N.Y.S.2d 938, 940 (1950); and Commonwealth ex rel. Flannery v. Sharp, 30 A.2d 810 (Pa. Super. 1943).

24. E.g., Odell v. Lutz, and Succession of Reiss, supra.

25. E.g., Succession of Reiss, 46 La. Ann. 347, 15 So. 151 (1894); and Commonwealth ex rel. Flannery v. Sharp, supra.'

26. See 1966 N.Y. Stage legis. Annual 14.

26A. A number of other states have bills pending which would provide for grandparents' visitation, among which are Alabama, Georgia, Nebraska, Virginia and West Virginia.

27. Laws 1966, ch. 631 § 1; amended laws 1975, ch. 431, § 1.

28. See Geri v. Fanto, 79 Misc. 2d 947, 361 N.Y.S.2d 984 (Fam. Ct. 1974).

29. Laws 1975, ch. 431, § 1, effective July 1975.

30. Okl. Stat. Ann. § 60.16.

31. Calif. Civil Code 197.5 subdiv. c, stipulates that visitation rights shall not be awarded if the child has been adopted by a person other than a stepparent or grandparent.

32. Minn. Stats. Ann. § 257.022 subdiv. 3 provides that visitation shall not be granted if the child has been adopted by one other than a stepparent or grandparent. Under both the Minnesota statutes a prior award of visitation rights to grandparents is automatically terminated if the child subsequently is adopted by one other than a stepparent or grandparent.

33. The conflicting cases are cited in Graziano v. Davis, 50 Ohio App. 2d 83, 361 N.E.2d 525, 529 (1976), which held that an adoption by relative did not terminate grandparent visitation. Cases from Kansas, Louisiana, New York, and Texas have held that adoption, even by a relative, terminates visitation, whereas California, New York, and New Jersey have held visitation rights survive.

34. For example, the statutes in California and Minnesota, supra notes 31 and 32.

35. H.B. 971 has been introduced in the Louisiana legislature and it provides that grandparents may seek visitation rights with adopted children. In Oklahoma, the law has been amended by Laws 1978, ch. 71, to permit visitation with grandparents under certain circumstances after adoption.

36. Calif. Civ. Code § 4601.

37. Conn. Gen. Stats. Ann. § 46-42.

38. Hawaii Rev. Stats. § 571-46 subdiv. 7.

39. Ohio Rev. Code § 3109.11.

40. Minn. Stat. Ann. § 257.022.

41. Idaho Rev. Code § 32.1008.

42. See Goldstein, Freud, and Solnit, Beyond the Best Interests of the Child, Chap. 3 (1973).

43. See Re Reimenschneider, 164 N.W. 736 (Iowa 1917), where a maternal aunt was apointed guardian of an orphan over the opposition of grandparents. See also Adoption of Jackson, 201 Wis. 642, 321 N.W. 158 (1930), where custody of an orphan was awarded to a paternal aunt and uncle rather than grandparents. Compare Pruitt v. Key, 281 Ala. 433,

203 So. 2d 450, 30 A.L.R.3d 284 (1967), where four children were awarded to the custody of paternal grandparents, rather than a maternal aunt and uncle, after the father of the children had been sentenced to life imprisonment for killing the mother. In Kouris v. Lunn, 257 Iowa 1267, 136 N.W.2d 502 (1965), a three-year-old boy was awarded to his maternal great-aunt, rather than to his mother or maternal grandmother.

44. In Holmes v. Derrig, 127 Iowa 625, 103 N.W. 973 (1905), a three-year-old boy was awarded to his grandparent rather than to his stepfather or paternal uncle. For cases involving other relatives, see Annot., 30 A.L.R.3d 290,352.

45. 177 P.2d 628 (Cal. App. 1947).

46. See In re Fahlman, 84 Cal. App. 248, 257 P. 893 (1927); Kentera v. Kentera, 66 Cal. App. 2d 373, 152 P.2d 238 (1944).

47. 177 P.2d at 629.

48. See In re Marriage of Meier, 51 Cal. Rptr. 822 (1975), which discusses the first California statute and notes that an exception was made where parties stipulated as to visitation as in Bookstein, 7 Cal. App. 3d 219, 86 Cal. Rptr. 495 (1970).

49. Id.

50. 275 Cal. App. 2d 912, 80 Cal. Rptr. 432 (1969).

51. 53 Cal. App. 3d 1019, 126 Cal. Rptr. 51 (1975).

52. 44 Cal. App. 3d 687, 118 Cal. Rptr. 804 (1975).

53. 40 A.D.2d 296, 339 N.Y.S.2d 708 (4th Dept. 1973).

54. 54 Misc. 2d 843, 233, N.Y.S.2d 483 (Nassau Co. 1967).

55. 44 Cal. App. 3d 687, 118 Cal. Rptr. 804 (1975).

56. 113 Cal. App. 2d 531, 248 P.2d 425 (1952).

57. 7 Cal. App. 3d 219, 86 Cal Rptr. 495 (1970).

58. 66 N.J. 426, 332 A.2d 199 (1975).

59. 50 Ohio App. 2d 83, 361 N.E.2d 525 (1976).

60. Browning v. Tarwater, 215 Kan. 501, 524 P.2d 1135 (1974).

61. Smith v. Trosclair, 303 So. 2d 926 (La. App. 1974).

62. Deweese v. Crawford, 520 S.W.2d 522 (Tex. Civ. App. 1975).

63. People ex rel. Levine v. Rado, 54 Misc. 2d 843, 283 N.Y.S.2d 483 (1967).

64. For example, see In the Matter of Adoption of the Child by M. 140, N.J. Super. 91, 355 A.2d 211 (1976).

65. 150 N.J. Super. 509, 376, A.2d 191 (1977).

66. In the Matter of Adoption of a Child by M, 140 N.J. Super. 91, 355 A.2d 211 (1976).

67. N.J. Stat. Ann. § 9:2-7.1.

68. Apparently, there is no case which has been reported where there was such an accumulation of visitation rights that imperiled the welfare of the child. See Note, Statutory Visitation of Grandparents: One Step Closer to the Best Interests of the Child, 26 Cath. Univ. L. Rev. 387, at 397 (1977).

69. For example, see Odell v. Lutz, 177 P.2d 628 (Cal. App. 1947).

70. See Note, Visitation Rights of a Grandparent Over the Objection of the Parent: The Best Interests of the Child, 15 J. Fam. Law 51, 60 et seq. (1976-7). See also Scranton v. Hutter, 40 A.D.2d 296, 339, N.Y.S.2d 708 (4th Dept. 1973); and Mimkon v. Ford, 66 N.J. 426, 332 A.2d 199 (1975).

71. 4 F.L.R. 2397 (Pa. Super. 1978) (April 13, 1978).

72. 192 Pa. Super. 1, 159 A.2d 70 (1960).

73. Id. 192 Pa. Super. at 2, 159, A.2d at 71.

74. 170 Pa. Super. 254, 85 A2d 686 (1952).

75. Evans v. Lane, 8 Ga. App. 826, 70 S.E. 603 (1911).

76. Maddox v. Maddox, 174 Md. 470, 199 A. 507 (1938). See also Lo Presti v. Lo Presti, 40 N.Y.2d 522, 387 N.Y.S.2d 412, 355, N.E.2d 372 (1976), on remand, 54 A.D.2d 582, 387 N.Y.S.2d 153 (2d Dept. 1976).

77. 44 Cal. App. 3d 687, 118 Cal. Rptr. 804 (1975).

78. 113 Cal. App. 3d 531, 248 P.2d 425 (1925).

79. See Goldstein, Freud, and Solnit, Beyond the Best Interests of the Child 38 (1973).

80. See Pierce v. Yerkovich. 80 Misc. 2d 613, 363 N.Y.S.2d 403 (Fam. Ct. Ulster Co. 1974).

81. See Note, Visitation Rights of a Grandparent Over the Objection of a Parent: The Best Interests of the Child, 15 J. Fam. Law 51, 61 (1976-77); and Lo Presti v. Lo Presti, op. cit. supra note 101.

82. 151 Pa. Supr. 612, 30 A.2d 810 (1943).

83. 47 Ohio App. 2d 238, 353 N.E. 2d 884 (1975).

84. 330 Ill. App. 506, 71 N.E.2d 920 (1947).

85. 55 A.D.2d 953, 391 N.Y.S.2d 152 (2d Dept. 1977).

86. See Commonwealth ex rel. Flannery v. Sharp, 151 Pa. Super. 612, 30 A.2d 810 (1943); and Kay v. Kay, 51 Ohio Op. 434, 65 Ohio L. Sbs. 472, 112 N.E.2d 562 (1953).

87. 113 Cal. App. 2d 531, 248 P.2d 425 (1953).

88. See Note, Statutory Visitation Rights of Grandparents: One Step Closer to the Best Interests of the Child, 26 Cath. Univ. L. Rev. 387, 391 (1977).

89. 196 Pa. Super 46, 173 A.2d 650 (1961) assumed that the grandmother had no legal relationship with the child and functioned as a distant third party because the child had been adopted by the daughter and son-in-law of the grandparents.

90. See Annot., 25 A.L.R.3d 7; Annot., 29 A.L.R.3d 366; Annot., 30 A.L.R.3d 290; Annot., 31 A.L.R.3d 1187.

91. See Note, Statutory Visitation Rights for Grandparents: One Step Closer to the Best Interests of the Child, 26 Cath. Univ. L. Rev. 387, 289 (1977); Kay v. Kay, 51 Ohio Op. 434, 112 N.E.2d 562 (1953); and People ex rel. Schachter v. Kahn, 241 App. Div. 686, 269 N.Y.S. 173 (2d Dept. 1934).

92. For example, see People ex rel. Scarpetta v. Spence-Chapin Adoption Services, 28 N.Y.2d 185, 321 N.Y.S.2d 65, 269 N.E.2d 787, cert. denied, 404 U.S.805 (1971), where the New York court presumed that the best interests of a child would be furthered by its return to its natural mother although she had placed the child for adoption.

93. See Foster and Freed, Life With Father, 1978, 11 Fam. L.Q. 321, 325 et seq. (1978).

94. Unites States v. Green, 26 F. Cas. (D.R.I. 1824) No. 15,256.

95. For example, see King v. De Manneville, 3 East 221, 102 Eng. Rep. 1054 (1800); Ex parte Skinner, 9 Moore 278 (1824); and People ex rel. Olmstead v. Olmstead, 27 Barb. 9 (N.Y. 1857).

96. Obrecht v. McClane, 256 S.W.2d 955 (Tex. Civ. App. 1953); Jones v. Jones, 349 Mass. 259, 207 N.E.2d 922 (1965).

97. Succession of Simkin, 164 La. 223, 113 So. 825 (1927); Hesse v. Ashurst, 468 P.2d 343 (Nevada 1970); Application of Williams, 161 Neb. 686, 74 N.W.2d 543 (1956).

98. Osterholt v. Osterholt, 173 Neb. 683, 114 N.W.2d 734 (1962); Perkins v. Courson, 219 Ga. 611, 135 S.E.2d 388 (1964); Yancey v. Watson, 217 Ga. 215, 121 S.E.2d 772 (1961).

99. Alingh v. Alingh, 259 Iowa 219, 144 N.W.2d 134 (1966); Application of Vallemont, 182 Kan. 334, 321 P.2d 190 (1958).

100. State ex rel. Obrecht v. McClane, 256 S.W.2d 955 (Tex. Civ. App. 1953); Smith v. Jones, 275 Ala. 148, 153 So. 2d 226 (1963).

101. Alingh v. Alingh, 259 Iowa 219, 144 N.W.2d 134 (1956). Rothman v. Jewish Child Care Ass'n, N.Y.L.J. Nov. 1, 1972, p. 17, Cols. 2-4 (N.Y. Co., Nadel, J.).

102. Conley v. Walden, 533 P.2d 955 (Mont. 1975); State v. Blanco, 177 Nev. 149, 128 N.W.2d 615 (1964).

103. Bennett v. Jeffreys, 40 N.Y.2d 543, 387 N.Y.S.2d 821, 356 N.E.2d 277 (1976).

104. See Annot., 31 A.L.R.3d 1187, at 1196.

105. E.g., Mimkon v. Ford, 66 N.J. 426, 332 A.2d 199 (1975); Roquemore v. Roquemore, 275 Cal. App. 2d 912, 80 Cal. Rptr. 432 (1969); Scranton v. Hutter, 40 A.D.2d 296, 339 N.Y.S.2d 708 (4th Dept. 1973).

106. Bennett v. Clemens, 196 S.E.2d 842 (Ga. 1973). Compare Dieringer v. Heiney, 10 Ore. App. 345, 497 P.2d 1201 (1972).

107. 258 Iowa 1390, 140 N.W.2d 152, cert. denied, 385 U.S.949 (1966).

108. For an example of poor case work, see In re Rinker, 117 A.2d 780 (Pa. Super. 1955).

109. See Foster and Freed, Life With Father: 1978, 11 Fam. L.Q. 321, 325 et seq. (1978).

110. Levy v. Levy, N.Y.L.J., Jan, 29, 1976, p. 11, col. 3; p. 12, cols 1–6 (Co., J.); Lyritzis v. Lyritzis, 55 A.D.2d 946, 391 N.Y.S.2d 133 (2d Dept. 1977); Perotti v. Perotti, 355 N.Y.S.2d 68 (Sup. Ct., Queens Co., 1974).

111. See Pruitt v. Key, 281 Ala. 433, 203 So. 2d 450 (1967); and Brannan v. Brannan, 284 So. 2d 701 (Fla. App. 1973).

112. See op. cit. supra note 105.

113. 238 Ga. 374, 233 S.E.2d 353 (1977).

114. For example, Commonwealth ex rel. Graham v. Graham, 367 Pa. 553, 80 A.2d 829 (1951). See also Lippincott v. Lippincott, 97 N.J. Eq. 517, 128 A. 254, affirming 96 N.J. Eq. 260, 124 A. 532 (1924), which involved two sets of contending grandparents.

115. Annot., 25 A.L.R.3d 7,21.

116. Sass v. Sass, 246 Wis. 272, 16 N.W.2d 829 (1944).

117. Armstrong v. Manzo, 380 U.S. 545 (1965). See also Alsager v. District Court, 545 F.2d 1137 (8th Cir. 1976).

118. See dissenting opinion in Forbes v. Warren, 184 Miss. 526, 186 So. 325 (1939). Of course, if the best interests of the child require placement elsewhere, no constitutional issue is raised. See State ex rel. Cochrane v. Blanco, 177 Neb. 149, 128 N.W.2d 615 (1964).

119. See Alsager v. District Court, 545 F.2d 1137 (8th Cir. 1976), and Armstrong v. Manzo, 380 U.S. 545 (1965).

120. 321 U.S. 148 (1944).

121. 40 N.Y.2d 522, 387 N.Y.S.2d 412, 355 N.E.2d 372 (1976).

THE ECONOMIC CHOICE IN DIVORCE: EXTENDED OR BLENDED FAMILY?

Walter D. Johnson
Michael H. Minton

ABSTRACT. The creation of traditional family patterns and the transformation of these patterns into stereotypical nuclear study models has spawned a prolific amount of literature on individual happiness, psychological gratification and emotional self-sufficiency. The fragmentation of these family models through divorce has resulted in a breakdown of family function and a disassociation of its members.

While some attention has been paid to the economic impact of divorce on the nuclear family, little concern has been shown regarding the economic ramifications on the post-divorce family unit. It is hypothesized that in the post-divorce period, the nuclear has been reshaped or reformed into an extended family. The dissolution-fragmentation process changes the environment in which the family continues to function.

It is this extended family and the environment which sustains it that presents the focus of our inquiry. Although we do not disagree that the nuclear family is the predominant model as established by former study and literature, the dissolution process is, in fact, the procreator of another model—the extended family steps in as a surrogate protector, providing the environment (continuum) for the continuing existence of its offspring.

Walter D. Johnson, PhD, is Head of the Family Research Section of the Illinois Legislative Studies Center at Sangamon State University in Springfield, Illinois. He is a legal consultant in the area of financial negotiation of marital settlement agreements and serves on the Editorial Board of the *Journal of Divorce*. Michael H. Minton, JD, is an attorney-at-law in the State of Illinois specializing in matrimonial law. He is a partner in the Chicago based law firm of Facchini and Minton.

An acknowledgement of the extended family and recognition of the surrogate role it plays in the post-divorce environment belies the assertion that divorce is the death knell for the Family. The focus on the nuclear family to the exclusion of any other form of family existence has largely obscured, if not ignored, a social and economic reality, namely that families continue to function outside of marriage and after divorce. In the divorce process a family is said to collapse, when in reality it expands. Although the nuclear family model may shatter, the family heals itself by reaching out and expanding to meet its new needs. This expansion—the extended family—has a profound contemporary influence on its members.

To forecast the future of the blended family is premature. To compare the stamina of the nuclear family to the blended family is not yet possible. To question what makes a family strong, what enables it to endure, and how it continues to survive, are our topics of discussion. For those who "wrap themselves in the cloth of family," the inquiry must continue.

The overwhelming preoccupation with the nuclear family during the first half of the Twentieth Century resulted in such a narrow conceptualization of family and kinship that many important extended family relationships became obscured. Because the nuclear model was regarded as the natural family paradigm, necessary for a stable social structure, deviations from this norm implied failure of the family as an institution. Since the family was the basic unit of our social structure this failure was to be avoided if at all possible.

A clear example of this attitude is found in the policies, both social and legal, which prevailed regarding divorce. The rules and guidelines governing the household unit were geared towards inhibiting divorce. The common family concept presupposed that each nuclear family lived as an independent household. Both parents had to be present in the home to fulfill their roles if the family were to function properly. The marital bond had to remain intact or the functional relationships, which supposedly existed mostly between parents and children would cease to be performed. The prevalence of this thought pattern was clearly evident in the fault-based system of divorce which predominated in the various states up through the past decade.

The advent of no-fault, as personified in the Uniform Marriage and Divorce Act, has removed the socio-psychological admonishments which grounds for divorce carried, but it has not provided a basis for recognizing that many family functions can and must be met outside the immediate parent/child relationship of the nuclear model, and that other family forms may indeed be viable. Divorce, in fact, has been a major contributor to the creation of these new family forms.

The most obvious example of this social processing is the single-parent family. The single-parent household has become the most rapidly increasing family form in America today. It accounts for almost 20 percent of the 57 million families in America. Single parenthood is most often not a choice, but a condition: a condition perpetrated on divorcing families through the economic impacting of our legal system. Single parenthood is an intermediate step between the nuclear family model and the families of the future.

Currently, only one out of four of the 80 percent classified as two-parent families fits the traditional nuclear mold of breadwinner-home-maker-children. Increasingly it is apparent that while the upswing in divorce is the primary reason for the growth of single-parent households, the majority of single parents will remarry or reenter an altered form of the two-adult model. U.S. Census Bureau estimates indicate that 40 percent of the marriages now being formed will end in divorce. Three out of four of those divorcing will remarry and reenter the two-parent model. Of those who do remarry, 21 percent will do so within a year of their divorce and 75 percent before the end of the fifth year. In this context, single-parenthood becomes a transitional state.

Given the psychological trauma of divorce, questions arise as to why these individuals move back into a marital relationship and why so quickly. While there is no single answer, an overriding factor is the economic deprivation occasioned by divorce. Most individuals simply do not have the resources to remain divorced. That they survive at all in single parenthood is often due to the assistance they receive from their extended family. For many of these individuals support from the extended family is a logical extension of the support network which existed in their marriage.

Marriage and the Extended Family

Contrary to what the nuclear model would imply, the economic ties of the extended family, although shifting in form, have remained very much intact during the post-war period. The primary facilitator of this relationship has been the cost of acquiring and maintaining the much publicized middle class social standing. Parental experiences in the 1930's coupled with the instability of the war years gave rise to a mass social movement directed toward the attainment of monetary security and status. Preoccupation with a standard of living was reinforced by the unprecedented economic growth of the American economy. As the composition of the labor force shifted from the discernible white-collar/ blue-collar structure of the 1940's and 50's to the service-dominated occupations of the 70's, technical skills and training took on new importance. This change demanded mass involvement of the populace in post-secondary education. Parental financing of their children's education became one of the most significant contributions of the extended family to the current generation of adults. Higher education meant more than job security; it meant suburbia, two-car garages, color televisions and radar ranges. Attaining the "good life" became more than socially acceptable. It became a dominating objective.

The acceleration in material needs led to an expectational level which usually far exceeded the actual financial resource base of most young adults attaining marital age in the 1960's and 70's. But, as was the case with education, more and more parents could be counted on for economic assistance when their children decided to marry or set up a household. This allowed many young couples to bypass a good portion of the financial struggle that had marked their parents' lives. While children moved into their own homes and went on to new careers, their physical separation from parents did not remove the strong family links grounded in economic support. The extended family continued, less visible but nonetheless extremely important.

These high expectational levels were shared by those forming families whose parents were not in a position to provide economic resources. The rise in material expectations was not simply a middle class phenomenon, but was the driving force behind the creation of a middle class. The installment plan allowed families not funded by parents to emulate their contemporaries. Credit became a substitute for the economic resources of the extended family.

Thus, the economic contributions of others formed an integral step in the construction of many of the nuclear families of this generation. In turn, as these families began to dissolve through divorce, these instruments and interests rekindled extended family involvement.

The Dissolution Process

The aspiration for economic security, so important in the marital relationship, is also a focal point in the divorce process. Years of measuring relative well-being in monetary terms results in the majority of divorces evolving into perceived struggles for economic survival. But the spoils of marriage are not simply the product of the involved spouses. By virtue of their contribution to the marital unit, members of the extended family in their protective role reenter to argue for or protect various investments in the nuclear relationship as well as to assist their offspring. As a result, economic apportionment and the assignment of financial responsibility become emotionally laden and explosive issues, necessitating skillful negotiation and an ability to foresee future circumstances.

The Attorney

Disassembling the nuclear unit requires that the loosely defined parameters of the marriage vows be replaced with the comprehensive provisions of a divorce contract or marital settlement agreement. One of the most important decisions to be made in preparation for these negotiations involves choosing an attorney to represent the interests of these varied concerns. Obviously matrimonial attorneys are more than facilitators of procedural events. They are the protectors and pursuers of economic justice as perceived by these interested parties. As such, lawyers become surrogate members of the extended family. The choice of an attorney is in fact likely to be heavily influenced by the extended family. Most individuals lack familiarity with the legal community and will seek out referrals from their family or close friends. The extended family may, indeed, find itself involved in the hiring of the attorney.

Legal recognition of the dissolution can entail substantial expenditure depending on the size of the estate, the individual's income, the number of children, and, most importantly, the degree of anger and frustration between the spouses. The major expense in this process is representation. Given the expenditure debt pattern that most families have fallen into and the fact that three quarters of all divorce actions are filed by women who are least likely to control the economic resources of the family, legal fees become an immediate issue (Plateris, 1973; W. Johnson, 1979). Faced with this dilemma, most clients, and particularly women, end up borrowing funds from relatives or friends to pay their attorney's retainer. Thus, the extended family plays a pivotal role in initiating the divorce process.

Marital Settlement Agreements

Once legal representation is obtained, economic concerns are shifted toward the division of accumulated wealth and future security. Two key determinative factors enter into this process: the identification of what is and is not marital property, and the assignment of custody where children are involved (W. Johnson, 1978; Minton and W. Johnson, 1979). Both involve interests of the extended family.

As previously indicated, the question of what constitutes marital property has taken on added significance in recent years due to the increased contributions of the extended family to the establishment of the household in which the new marrieds will live. These contributions may have been made prior to the actual marriage or during its existence. Invariably, those extended family members who made a specific contribution argue for its disposition in favor of their kin. The most prevalent example is the marital home which may have been purchased from relatives at a reduced price or may have been purchased with money supplied by parents. Stocks, bonds, and other financial investments made on behalf of their divorcing adult children or given during the course of the marriage are also becoming prevalent issues in settlement negotiations. In terms of absolute number, the most often encountered item of extended family interest is the family heirloom which has been passed down from generation to generation. The necessity of determination in these areas has resulted in the increased appearance in the legal literature of guidelines for deciphering what is and is not marital property (Auerbach, 1979).

With regard to the custodial issue, formulas and guidelines for the adjustment of property, support, and maintenance, as set forth by statute and/or case decisions, are increasingly based upon child placement. This is clearly evidenced in the Topical provisions set forth in the Uniform Marriage and Divorce Act (UMDA).

The trial or settlement of a dissolution case attaches significant economic rewards to the party obtaining custody of the child or children. The economic see-saw experienced during the marriage halts dramatically when the award of custody is determined. If the wife receives custody, she obtains support for the child, occupancy of a home for the child, medical and educational benefits for the child, and perhaps maintenance for herself to stay with the child. If the husband receives custody, he is free of monetary payments to his estranged spouse as well as control over the time and amount of payments made in relation to his child. Additional benefits include the probable freedom from maintenance payments, tax deductions, and the occupancy of the home or at least an immediate remuneration from its sale.

These outcomes influence decidedly the economic future of not only the disassociating nuclear family members but also their relationships with and financial demands upon the extended family network. Unfortunately the breadth of control that the marital settlement agreement exercises and the repercussions it is likely to cause are most often not realized until after its finalization. Compounding the problem is the decided lack of support provided by the structure which governed the dissolution. With the signing of the divorce decree the legal system, for all practical purposes, ends its involvement with the family form it has helped to create.

The process with the paraphernalia of courtroom, lawyers and judges, and their role in the division of one's home, the allocation of income, and the taking of children, creates an environment over which the system itself quickly loses control. It establishes directions and guidelines for which it has neither the ability nor the intention of overseeing. Whereas in the natural-family paradigm which formerly governed marital law, marriage and divorce were means to an end, under the legal-family paradigm they have become ends in themselves (Farber, 1973). Once the divorce is granted the legal process shifts functional responsibility back to the individuals and/or the extended family (W. Johnson, 1976). This is evident clearly in the post-divorce environment of the single-parent family.

The Single-Parent Family

For men, the assignment of the major portion of marital property to their former wives (as the custodial parent) normally places them at a distinct financial disadvantage and often perpetuates the idea that visitation parenting is temporary parenting. It fails to recognize that divorce creates the need for two homes where children can visit in comfort and where parents can continue to relate to their children. Aside from adding to the potential hostility between parents, it forces the non-custodial parent to assume the cost of restructuring the parent-child relationship. In many instances, this cannot be done without financial assistance from the former husband's family, which not only involves grandparents and relatives in the financial aspects of the divorce but is quite likely to increase the hostility level between former in-laws.

On the other side, divorce is likely to create severe hardships for the domestic homemaker. This is particularly true for those women who choose the traditional housewife-mother role. Historically alimony, or maintenance as it is now termed, was designed to protect these women. Unfortunately, this major financial consideration has come close to disappearing in contemporary society. The increased entrance of women into the labor force has been the primary reason for this alteration. Maintenance is only infrequently given and support allocations tend more and more to utilize the income differential principle. The amount of the support allocation no longer depends entirely on the husband's income but on the difference between the potential earning capacity of the mother and the resources needed to maintain an adequate level of living for the children. (See the Maintenance and Support Section of the UMDA.) Less than 5 percent of all settlement agreements now provide for maintenance payments. (Information collected from a sample of 8,600 divorced families being processed at this writing by W. Johnson.) These women must now seek financial support from outside the nuclear household through their own employment, from their extended family, or from social service programs.

Employment

The increased employment of women in the post-war period and the preeminence of child support have been the major factors in the demise of maintenance. Between 1950 and 1975, the civilian labor force grew by almost 50 percent, from 62.2 million to 92.6 million. Approximately two-thirds of this growth was accounted for by the increased employment of women. By 1975, 37.0 million or 40 percent of the civilian labor force were women. (Sum, 1977)

Even in those instances where women are not employed, the courts are now likely to disallow maintenance on the grounds of their potential employability. However, there is a real danger of confusing potential with actual resource availability. While employment opportunities for women have risen significantly over the past thirty years, women still earn substantially less than men.

Income

In 1977 the median income of families headed by women was only $7,765 or 43 percent of that of husband-wife families. (B. Johnson, 1978) Even in those traditional husband-wife families where the husband was the only wage earner, median income was twice that of families headed by women. This disparity is even greater when measured against husband-wife families in which both spouses worked. Income in these families is almost triple that of female-headed families.

The lower income potential for these women serves to increase the importance of their employment as evidenced in their labor force participation rates. In 1978, 77.6 percent of the divorced female family heads were employed compared to only 40.8 percent of the women in two-parent households. Divorcees are also more likely to work all year and to work full time. Interestingly, U.S. Labor Department surveys have found that the major reason given by married women for their aversion to full-time employment is the presence of children and/or other family responsibilities. Divorced mothers on the other hand are forced into the labor market for these very same reasons.

Children

The existence of children in these single-parent households adds considerably to the economic pressures experienced by these families and increases the need for extended family involvement. Invariably, income gaps are wider between those families with children and those without. In addition, those families headed by a woman as a result of divorce contain a disproportionately high share of children. Over 70 percent of divorced female heads of households are between the ages of 18 and 44, the most probable age group for having young children at home. Almost 8 percent are under 24 and 33 percent are between 25 and 34. (Bureau of Labor Statistics, 1976) These groups are the most likely to have preschool and elementary-grade children, necessitating full or part-time child care if the mother works. This situation has resulted in an increase in both the absolute number of children involved in divorce and their rate per 1000 children in recent years. (W. Johnson, 1979) One out of every six children now lives in a single-parent family and, more alarmingly, it is estimated that two of every five born in the 1970's will spend at least five of these childhood years in such a household. The combination of children and low earning potential results in a reduction in the available income per individual family member in those units which are divorce created, from $4,500 to $2,500, a substantial reduction by any standard.

Child Support

Child support awards are supposedly designed to mitigate this difference transferring income to the household responsible for the economic support of the children. However the granting of these awards and their payment have become two distinctly different issues.

Ideally, the divorce contract provides the guidelines for a new relationship, particularly with regard to children and finances. In reality, it provides the mechanism for continued warfare. One of the most common weapons is the withholding of support payments. Unfortunately, the severity of this has been downplayed through the assumption that it occurs only infrequently and/or only in the lower socio-economic classes. Empirical study, however, indicates that nonpayment of child support is a major problem.

The degree of noncompliance with court-ordered child support was first examined by Eckhardt (1968). Utilizing a group of Wisconsin divorces granted in 1955 it was found that only 38 percent of the fathers ordered to pay child support were in full compliance at the end of the first year. At the end of five years, the percentage had dropped to 19. While a few partially complied during the time-frame of the study, the majority of fathers stopped paying completely after the first year.

Two more recent studies in Illinois provide essentially the same picture. (W. Johnson, 1979) The first, examining divorces granted in a seven-county area in 1965, found that full compliance ranged from a mere 53 percent in the year the divorce was granted to a low of 21 percent 11 years later. A second examination of these same counties utilizing divorces granted in 1970 indicated an even higher default rate. Only 43 percent complied with the support provision in the first year. Full compliance dropped to 28 percent by the end of the second year and to 19 percent by the end of the sixth year.

All three studies exhibited the same basic traits. First, it was always the mother who received custody and the father who was liable for payment. Second, a substantial portion of those ordered to pay child support immediately disregarded their obligation. In some Illinois counties, as high as 45 percent of the fathers never made a single payment. Third, of those who originally complied with the court order, three-fourths stopped between the first and fourth years. In effect, the payer would engage in a testing process whereby a payment would be skipped and in the absence of legal action, the procedure would be repeated in a few months. As the periodic misses went unchallenged, their frequency increased until payment ceased completely.

A comparison of the two Illinois samples also indicated that not only has noncompliance increased but that enforcement processes are basically non-existent. The burden of enforcement is shifted from the court which originally made the award to the custodial parent. In order to force compliance, the recipient usually has to hire an attorney at her own expense. However, the absence of support quite likely places her in a marginal income situation which precludes paying a retainer. If she has the funds to institute an action, the outcome is normally a court reprimand and an agreement by the defaulting payer to comply. Once adjudicated, the process is likely to be repeated over and over again until the custodial parent gives up.

Observations

When situational need and resource availability are measured against one another, single-parent families created through divorce are quite likely to suffer from severe economic deprivation. This is particularly true for families headed by women.

The cost of family maintenance under comparable circumstances depreciates very little with the exit of one of the spouses. Housing, transportation and educational expenditures remain virtually unchanged. Food, utilities, clothing and medical costs decline but less than proportionately due to the reversed effect of economics of scale. Those reductions that do occur tend to be offset by increased spending on child care and services formerly performed by the disassociated spouse. On the other side of the ledger income falls off sharply, maintenance is infrequently awarded, and child support payments tend to be sporadic or non-existent. Given this situation the choice is limited: poverty or near-poverty, continued support by the extended family or movement back into the two-parent model.

Conclusions

Despite the prevalence of marital disruption in the United States relatively little research is available on how extended family assistance systems function after divorce. This is particularly true in the realm of economic support. It is evident that this support is needed in light of the data on the declining economic status of the family after divorce. It is also clear that financial support from the extended family plays an integral role in the formative stages of the marriage, its continuation, and its legal dissolution. There is some evidence, however, that the economic support available after divorce is either not of sufficient size or duration to make single parenthood a viable family form in the long run for the majority of those who experience it.

The first indicator is the tremendous growth of participation in the federally funded Aid For Dependent Children programs administered by the various states. Skyrocketing costs of this program in the 1970's led the federal government to initiate programs, such as the Child Support Enforcement Act, geared towards at least partially forcing responsibility for family support back on to errant parents.

A second indicator of limitations on extended family financial support is the aforementioned movement of most divorcing individuals back into a marital relationship. The National Center for Health Statistics has reported that three-quarters of the approximately 6 million women in the United States in 1976 who were between the ages of 15 and 44 whose first marriage had ended in divorce had remarried. Thus while single-parenthood may be the fastest growing alternative to a two-parent family, relatively few individuals choose to remain in this situation. The resultant "blended family" has become the logical alternative for the growing number of disassociated families just as divorce itself became the alternative to marriage. While it is too early to forecast the future of the "blended family," its link to the resurgence of the extended family is clearly established. Whether the extended family is allowed to continue to reassert itself remains to be seen.

REFERENCES

Auerbach, Marshall J. "Property Considerations Upon Dissolution and Declaration of Invalidity." *Family Law Volume II*, Springfield, Illinois, Illinois Institute for Continuing Legal Education, 1979.

Bureau of Labor Statistics, U.S. Department of Commerce. *Women Who Head Families: A Socio-Economic Analysis*, Washington, D.C.: Government Printing Office, 1976.

Colletta, Nancy Donohue *Support Systems After Divorce: Incidence and Impact*. Unpublished Research Conducted at the Institute for Child Study, University of Maryland, 1977.

Eckhardt, Kenneth "Deviance, Visability and Legal Action: The Duty to Support." *Social Problems*, Volume 15, 1968.

Farber, Bernard *Family and Kinship in Modern Society*. Glenview, Illinois: Scott, Foresman and Company, 1973.

Glick, Paul and Norton, S. *Marrying, Divorcing and Living Together in the U.S. Today*. Washington, D.C.: Population Deference Bureau, 1977.

Grady, William R. *Remarriages of Women 15-44 Years of Age Whose First Marriage Ended in Divorce: United States, 1976*. Advance data from Vital & Health Statistics of the National Center for Health Statistics, No. 58, Feb. 14, 1980.

Grossman, Allyson Sherman "Divorced and Separated Women in the Labor Force—An Update." *Monthly Labor Review*, Volume 101, No. 10, October, 1978.

Johnson, Beverly L. "Marital and Family Characteristics of Workers 1970-1978." Special Labor Force Report No. 219. Bureau of Labor Statistics, U.S. Department of Labor, 1978.

Johnson, Walter D. "Divorce, Alimony, Support, and Custody: A Survey of Judges' Attitudes in One State." *The Family Law Reporter*, Volume 3, No. 2, 1976.

Johnson, Walter D. "The Economic Ramifications of Divorce," *Conciliation Court Review*. Volume 14, No. 1, Sept. 1976.

Johnson, Walter D. "Growing Pains in Child Support." *Illinois Issues*, Volume IV, No. 4, April, 1978.

Johnson, Walter D. *Policy Implications of Divorce Reform*. Springfield, Illinois, Illinois Legislative Studies Center, 1979.

Mayleas, Davidyne *Rewedded Bliss*. New York: Basic Books, 1977.

Minton, Michael H., and Johnson, Walter D. "The Use of Experts in Matrimonial Cases." *Illinois Family Law Volume II*, Springfield, Illinois: Illinois Institute for Continuing Legal Education, 1979.

Plateris, Alexander A. *100 Years of Marriage and Divorce Statistics*. U.S. Department of Health, Education and Welfare. Health Resources Administration Series 21, No. 24, Washington, D.C.: Government Printing Office, 1973.

Sum, Andrew M. "Female Labor Force Participation: Why Projections Have Been Too Low." *Monthly Labor Review*, July, 1977.

DIVORCE: A POTENTIAL GROWTH EXPERIENCE FOR THE EXTENDED FAMILY

Florence Kaslow

Ralph Hyatt

ABSTRACT. This article discusses some of the ways in which divorce, usually conceived of as a primarily negative and painful experience, can be turned to positive advantage, and have a beneficial impact on the divorcing person's extended family. The authors indicate that when the divorcing one copes well, his behavior serves as a model for handling difficulty well and diminishes others' fears about losses and embarking on new relationships. Also, such a major event causes repercussions in the interactions between family members, calling into play new attitudes and behavior patterns.

A Traumatic and Often Demeaning Process

The far reaching emotional impact and negative reverberations of separation and divorce have been repeatedly documented (Hunt and Hunt, 1977; Weiss, 1975; Epstein, 1974). Weiss (1975) has commented about the broken attachment of spouses in the following way:

Florence Kaslow, PhD, was formerly Dean and Professor at the Florida School of Professional Psychology in Miami, Florida. She is Editor of the *Journal of Marital and Family Therapy*, on the Editorial Board of *Journal of Divorce* and other Journals, author of many books and articles in marital, family and divorce therapy and has guest lectured on these subjects throughout the world. Ralph Hyatt, EdD, is Chairman and Professor in the Department of Psychology at St. Joseph's College in Philadelphia. He is the Editor of the Psychology Section of *USA Today* and author of "Before you Marry Again," and numerous other books and articles.

Once developed, attachment seems to persist. Even when marriages turn bad and the other components of love fade or turn into their opposites, attachment is likely to remain. The spouses resemble battered children in their feelings. They may be angry, even furious, with one another; they may hate one another for past injuries and fear one another's next outburst of rage. (p. 14)

Husband and wife may attempt to retaliate, seek immediate retribution or harbor hidden desires for ultimate revenge to redress the anguish and abandonment.

Holmes and Rahe, in their 1967 Social Readjustment Rating Scale, placed divorce second only to death of a spouse as a stressful life event. Our observation is that sometimes divorce is more overwhelming since the rejection and perceived abandonment are more deliberate and perhaps more analogous to death when the spouse has committed suicide.

The analogy between divorce and death has perhaps been exaggerated. Yet, the observations of many clinicians testify to the strong probability of the occurrence of stages similar to the one's identified by Kubler-Ross (1969) in the process of the death of a loved one, that is: denial, anger, bargaining, depression, and resignation or acceptance as emotional landmarks, if not universal stages, in the experiences of those who divorce (Froiland and Hozman, 1977). The mourning process must be attended to so that healing of the emotional wounds can occur and some closure can be achieved before one is ready to engage in new trusting and meaningful relationships.

Whether one subscribes to Bohannan's (1973) six stations of divorce, Kessler's (1975) seven stage model, or Kaslow's (1980b) dialectic model, one finds commonalities in their formulations. Recuperation and re-equilibration seem to take about two years from the time the pre-divorce separation occurred. It is rare that a reactive depression, periods of self-pity and self-disparagement, rapid mood swings, tremendous ambivalence, withdrawal, crying jags, irritability, and uncontrollable verbal outpourings are not experienced and displayed during the process of separating and divorcing. Even temperamentally calm individuals fluctuate emotionally and at times feel and seem "crazy." It is important that their friends, relatives, colleagues and therapists recognize and handle these temporary reactions as "normal" and to be expected during this emotionally turbulent period. These affective sequelae of the marital disruption seem to be essential precursors to a new, often higher level of integration and functioning.

Legal machinations often escalate the fray, diminishing the two parties' sense of justice and rationality while heightening their manipulativeness and vituperativeness. Because legal entanglements generally tend to have a long range impact on the ex-couple, their children, and relatives, we believe therapist and attorney alike should encourage fairness and a humane concern for everyone involved, and that, whenever possible, interdisciplinary cooperation (Black and Joffee, 1978; Kaslow, 1980A; Steinberg, 1980) should be engaged in to foster an equitable settlement and contribute to the potential of divorce as a growth experience.

Out of Ashes, a Phoenix Arises

The strength of the human organism is reflected in one's ability to eventually "pick up the pieces" and reenter the world to resume the interrelated processes of living and loving—which typically imply growing. Therapists and other astute observers, including many divorcees, indicate that ultimately divorce may revive feelings of self-esteem, a knowledge of one's ability to cope and survive, and can contribute to a sense of inner peace and harmony. If, indeed, the analogy to death is valid, the discarded partner and terminated marriage may be remembered but are no longer vital to one's existence.

Just as the suffering experienced in the divorce process may well lay the groundwork for *growth* for the divorcing parties, so too may it for those who touch their lives like siblings, grandparents, stepchildren, aunts, uncles, and cousins.

Jourard (1962) states, "Growth of the self is a change in the way of experiencing the world and one's own being" (p. 18). He elucidates, "one can speak of growth only when the changes enhance the person's ability to cope with challenges in his existence." In a true sense the pain of the divorce process can potentially serve as an impetus for growth of the divorced individual as he/she seeks a new integration. This quest can illuminate the path for members of his/her extended family to alter their perceptions of divorce and the divorcing person; it can enable them to see the rewarding aspects of responding well to the challenge. In seeing the strengths and ability to fashion something better out of the chaos, members of the divorced person's extended family too may venture to reshape disappointing, outmoded life patterns.

Carl Rogers emphasizes the "self" as a central construct and believes that "the forward-moving tendency can only operate when the choices are clearly perceived and adequately symbolized" (Hall and Lindsey, 1976,

p. 287). Rogers refers to the self-actualized person as "fully functioning," with characteristics of openness to experience, congruence between sense of self and organismic qualities, and love of self and others. It is this inherent forward moving tendency and desire for self-realization that we identify with and attempt to enhance in therapy. As the divorced person becomes increasingly self actualizing, there is a radiating and contagious quality which seems to convey a permission to their loved ones to also break out of despondent ruts and seek to create a more fulfilling way of living.

Horney also discusses "self-realization," stating (1950, p. 17): "And that is why I speak of the *real self* as that central inner force, common to all human beings and yet unique in each, which is the deep source of growth." She indicates that for her, growth is "always meant in the sense presented here...that of free, healthy development in accordance with the potentials of one's generic and individual nature." Maslow (1962) contrasts the survival tendency with the actualizing tendency in each person. Although the former is powerful and ultimately necessary, it sets the stage for truly human motivation. Maslow alludes to growth characteristics of creativity, unselfish love and peak experiences.

A commonality among the aforementioned neo-Freudians and humanist theoreticians and practitioners is that self-fulfillment and growth can be cultivated and thrive, given a warm, positive, accepting, supportive atmosphere—in spite of early negative conditions and abrasive antecedent experiences Horney (1950) Maslow (1962) Jourard (1968). Despite the agonizing crush to one's self-esteem in divorce, in the aftermath there can be a rebirth of the "real self" and a redefinition of one's world. This can embrace persons in the extended family. As one changes in fundamental ways, their significant others are likely to react in new ways, so that changes in the established relational patterns occur for them too, freeing them to also embark upon a change process.

De Burger (1977) has reinforced this idea:

> In an optimistic view we could speculate that the turbulence and change associated with termination of an established relationship may be a prelude to personal growth—growth which may improve the potential for meaningful interpersonal relations (p. 549).

That such breakthroughs do occur in reality is further borne out in the work of Johnson (1977), Krantzler (1974) and Fisher (1974). They all offer testament to the positive potential inherent in divorce, based on their experiences in seeing and working with many single-again individuals.

The Process of Growth

There are two main ways in which growth takes place for the divorced person and impacts favorably on their extended family. First is the dual process of modeling and emulation. In essence, how the divorced person behaves during the metamorphosis becomes a model for other family members in how to deal with strained interpersonal relationships and major life crises. Charny (1980) asserts the efficacy of learning to deal with interpersonal polarities rather than trying to avoid them—since indeed, it is virtually impossible to avert conflict and confrontation. The mastery of the transitional tasks and the rebuilding of one's life in a productive and independent mode by the divorced person also stimulates growth possibilities in the lives of his/her significant others. The latter do not have to commiserate sadly with one who is too busy and vitally engaged in the process of living to sulk; instead they can attempt to emulate the divorced person's thrust toward a new, more dynamic way of creating one's life-space.

As family members observe and come to admire the divorcee's courage and ability to venture forth into new activities, possibly changing jobs and entering into new friendships, they may be motivated to express their admiration. This serves to re-enforce the new attitudes and behaviors in the divorced person. In return the divorced person's successful coping and adaptations can diminish the sense of family members that they would become immobilized were they to be confronted by divorce. The ability of such family members to find they can deal competently with life's transitions, be these loss of loved one's through death, the departure of children for college or jobs out of town, the relocation of parents or close friends to better climes, may lead them to understand and find a new blueprint in the divorced relative's personal triumph.

Furthermore, new mature relationships may be established between and among extended family members as a result of the divorce experience. Initially, the psychic upheaval may cause them to reach out toward the distraught person—offering to listen to or be with the person in whatever ways they are needed. This can lead to breaking down existing barriers to closeness and affection and allow for sharing of confidences and the deep rooted loyalties felt by various members of the divorced person's family of origin. Or, the converse might be true. Members of the extended family may have occasion to learn to respect the divorcee's need for privacy and aloneness; this can reverse a family ethos of over-intrusiveness. Out of these novel emergent situations, the altered perceptions which accrue can serve to create or enhance warm, sensitive feelings and mutual respect within the family.

Unfortunately, such sets of new relationships do not develop easily or rapidly. As Goode (1956) reflected, there is failure in our post-divorce institutional arrangements. Kinship and social structures for all kinds of support—material and emotional—are woefully inadequate. Despite spiralling divorce rates in the 25 years since Goode's work, a recent review of the literature on divorce indicates that although more clinicians do divorce therapy, self-help groups like Parents without Partners have emerged, and singles clubs and apartments have come into prominence, our society as a whole has not yet formulated ceremonies or developed viable social policies to aid the transition and adjustment of the newly divorced and their offspring (Kaslow, 1980a).

Nonetheless, the *potential* for positive family supports exists. We see this in the development of novel interpersonal relations and the convening of networks through family reunions or visits to one's family of origin (Bowen, 1979). After divorce and an "unraveling procedure" (Hyatt, 1977), which includes an investigation of previous relational patterns with the entire family, positive changes can evolve which enable the divorced person to resist a re-creation of the "status quo ante." Let us examine further these growth-potential processes.

Impact on Members of Extended Family

As the divorce process unfolds, members of the extended family "observe the behavior...and its response consequences." If the relationship between the former spouses was dismantled with a sense of humanness, it can be an important lesson for others in the family who had contemplated separation in their own relationship but were afraid of the aloneness, stigma or nastiness. Perhaps a cousin or sibling who was committed to an exclusive relationship with his "lover" (either cohabiting or "going steady"), and in a continuous embattled state, can now feel more confident in altering the relationship in an atmosphere of understanding and amicability. They are freed to take the plunge and experience new depths of emotional living in a more committed and permanent relationship or in terminating it to seek a more gratifying relationship.

Another by-product we have witnessed is that a grandmother, watching her granddaughter become involved in diverse activities may realize that, *without guilt*, she may join a "Golden Age" group at the YWCA—

to do arts and crafts, attend lectures, or make one-day trips to New York City—*without* her eighty-two year old husband who is bent upon keeping her dependently cooped up in their 3-room apartment to be his full-time "guardian." Just as her granddaughter could no longer find tranquility and meaning in her life by losing herself in the irrational demands of her husband (after making many attempts at discovering rational options and solutions), and had decided "there must be more to life than this," so grandmother despite her feelings of stress, now derives the strength from her granddaughter to select more rational and varied paths for her own existence.

Acts of abuse during and after divorce provide ample opportunity for aunts, uncles, cousins, siblings and other family members to provide warmth, nurturance and support. If power plays were a problem for family members prior to the divorce, these may now be relinquished along with other animosities, as more adult communication systems are established and mutual-reciprocal relationships given the space and fresh air needed to flourish.

Although the magnitude of the escalating divorce statistics represent a massive jolt to our traditional marriage style and reflect weakened social pressure for an irrevocable marital commitment in that it is currently psychologically and legally easier to obtain a divorce, it has simultaneously created the *opportunity* for those willing to take it to guiltlessly renew and reevaluate a relationship without the feeling of being forever locked into a futile interpersonal cul-de-sac. Observing the courage of an extended family member "making the move" can be the impetus for another to take action on a long dormant idea or aspiration to venture onto new terrain in any of a variety of areas of his or her life.

The potential for growth is also inherent in the changes induced in the relationship network among other family members as they seek to help one of their members recuperate from an at best difficult, and at worst, devastating experience. At first the support may be in the context of "rescue" for a family member in the throes of emotional drowning. All may pitch in to take up the slack left by the exiting spouse's departure; grandmother baby sitting or preparing meals and feeling a rekindled sense of usefulness, dad helping around the house as a valued Mr. Fix-It or being a temporary substitute coach at Little League, and everyone encouraging the person with their belief that he or she can and will "pull your act together," reassuring him or her that they are cherished and respected in and by the family. Hence, some of the feared isolation and loneliness does not materialize.

Thus, after survival, to follow Maslow's conception (1962), there can be growth for all concerned. Siblings, stepsibs, grandparents and other family members can be brought closer because of the common problems to be solved. The family as an intertwined system and network functions interdependently and its healing properties are thus mobilized. A new unity may result when a divorced child develops a healthier attitude towards a stepparent who has traveled through similar muddy waters or when a sibling, who grew up with strong rivalrous feelings, now becomes empathic to his/her "war-torn" sister. An uncle may gain new respect for his "lazy, no-good" nephew who has finally bravely taken charge of his life by releasing himself from a domineering, castrating, shrewish wife. Upon his reentering the family with his new status, the nephew may find that family members who previously have taken advantage of his passive, non-assertive stance will be less apt to do so again. As his new found assertiveness is accorded respect, it is reenforced and the old pattern is truncated.

Special Implications for Step Parents

When a child or stepchild divorces, an interesting upturn in self-esteem can occur in the parent and the step-parent spouses who had been previously divorced without working through the divorce experience. The scars of feelings of failure start to fade when another family member, especially a stepchild whom *they* perceived never accepted them by virtue of their "inability to make it with another person," experiences his/her own separation. It is not so much that "misery loves company" as the realization that divorce does not mean personal failure or a permanent blemish on one's interpersonal skills and will now be so understood by the "model child" who has learned the lesson first-hand. A rapprochement between the two generations becomes more possible as they share an intuitive level of "knowing" each other.

Stepparents may benefit significantly from the reverberations of the divorce of a stepchild. If there were lingering perceptions of failure such as "My divorce was mostly my fault—There must be something wrong with me!"; the new divorce exonerates them when they realize "I guess I'm not *that* terrible—it even happened to this person." In some ways, it evens the score and minimizes residual child-to-parent blame. There is a better feeling about self since *other* family members will now understand that it could happen to anyone. And, after all, since most divorced people marry again the thinking is likely to become, "she may *also* someday be

a stepparent *like I am.*'' Indeed, it may help erase the ''Wicked Stepmother'' myth. A stepparent who may have been perceived as cold and
hypocritical will now have the chance to be nurturing and understand-
ingly empathic.

The opportunity to discuss ''anger'' and ''guilt'' in regard to the
divorce situation can serve to allow stepparents and stepchildren to
assess these same emotions in regard to their feelings toward each other.
The divorced child, who may once have maintained the fantasy that only
the natural nuclear family is ''healthy,'' now will realize that stepparenting is *not* a pathological phenomenon; someday they too may embark on
this role. The finality of one's own divorce will make the realistic
acceptance of his/her parents' remarriage much more accessible.

These feelings and associated behaviors will often affect other siblings who may have harbored similar confusions and misconceptions
about the stepparent's involvement in their family since in our society
these roles are not clearly defined (Visher & Visher, 1979). It may also
clarify ambivalent feelings about the divorce and remarriage of their
parents, such as ''I guess my parents couldn't make it, just like my sister
couldn't. And I understand her need to split,'' (this has occurred in their
generation and thus is more easily identified with), ''and so I now
comprehend my folks need to do so, too.'' The sense of loss and betrayal
felt by children when their parents divorce is heightened when parents
remarry. It ends the fantasy that their parents will remarry each other and
the family be reunited. The new divorce in the next younger generation
may help reduce the consternation felt by them earlier when as children
they believed they were the provocation for the divorce of their parents.
They now at last may be free of the supposition that ''it was my fault.''
Stepsiblings are frequently understood more clearly by the divorced
person who generally becomes sensitive to *any* disrupted relationship
and its residuals. Loss, failure, hurt, anger, anxiety, and new definitions
of love now become *shared* experiences.

An interesting side effect often spins-off onto the parents in a remarriage when one of their children divorces. When the stepparent exhibits
patience and love to the divorced adult-child of his/her spouse, he/she
conveys the clear message that their partner is accepted fully and uncon-
ditionally. By her actions she says in effect, ''What is yours is mine and I
accept responsibility *with* you for *our* mutual concerns.'' At times
''counting'' (''I brought only one child to our marriage, you contributed
four!''), which starts to cause a cleavage in many relationships, is
reduced to its absurdity when his one child is divorced and becomes the

catalyst for the entire family to pull together and firmly offer support to one another. When a stepparent, especially a stepfather (since the male role in our society is just beginning to accept tenderness and warmth as part of its ideal characteristics) can show these emotions to his divorced stepdaughter, or can empathize with the uncertainties and turmoil of his divorced stepson, the entire family relational system will be markedly altered.

Special Implications for Children

So far, little mention has been made herein of children since they are the relatives of the divorcing couple who to date, have received the most attention in the literature. (See for example, Kelly and Wallerstein, 1977; Kessler and Bostwick, 1977; and Gardner, 1976). However, it is important to note here that they too take their cues from their parents and emulate much of their behavior. If the parent(s) become fixated at the divorce juncture, continuing to squabble and gripe, harbor animosities and see life as misery, then the children are likely to feel obliged to take care of their distraught parents to atone for the alleged misdeeds of the other spouse. They may get pulled into taking sides on a prolonged basis and may develop a view of marriage as an archaic institution to be assiduously avoided. On the other hand, if both parents refrain from disparaging their ex-partner, a person they once loved and with whom they conceived their child or children, and move on to lead a full and rich life, again or for the first time, which appropriately includes the children and a positive attitude toward a good marriage, then the children are free to explore their world and have one and hopefully two parent models of how to cope successfully with life's exigencies.

Conclusion

Growth is a natural human process which occurs optimally in an open atmosphere of support, acceptance, and encouragement. At times this atmosphere evolves from negative conditions when one person in a family system—including the extended family membership—gets into personal difficulties and requires the solid and devoted help of significant others. Interestingly, there is a reciprocal reaction so that all who are involved can potentially grow. Divorce can indeed create the energy, for the divorced person, as well as extended family members, to deal meaningfully with many issues; role expectations, power, anxiety, dependence, guilt, frustrations, commitments, losses, love and freedom. Few persons enter marriage with the anticipation of divorce (unless original motives are devious or pathological), but if it must occur, there are positive outcomes which may accrue between the divorced and extended family members.

To increase the probability of such outcomes it may be wise for professionals in the field to be conversant with the stages of the divorce process from a psycholegal perspective (Kaslow, 1980a), and to utilize a family systems orientation in divorce therapy and beyond—treating the individual, or couple as need be, and involving children, parents, siblings and remarriage families when necessary so all can help in the healing process and reap potential benefits.

BIBLIOGRAPHY

Bandura, Albert and Walters, Richard H. *Social Learning and Personality Development.* New York: Holt, Rinehart and Winston, 1963.

Black, Melvin and Joffee, Wendy. A lawyer/therapist team approach to divorce. *Conciliation Courts Review*, June 1978, *16*, (1), 1-5.

Bohannan, Paul. The six stations of divorce. In Lasswell, Marcia E. and Lasswell, Thomas E. (Eds), *Love, Marriage and Family: A Develomental Approach*, Illinois: Scott, Foresman, 1973.

Boszormenyi-Nagy, Ivan and Spark, Geraldine. *Invisible Loyalties: Reciprocity in Intergenerational Family Therapy.* New York: Harper and Row, 1973.

Bowen, Murray. *Family Therapy in Clinical Practice.* New York: Jason Aronson, 1978.

Charny, Israel W. Why are so many (if not really all) people and families disturbed. *Journal of Marital and Family Therapy*, 1980, *6*, (1), 37-47.

Coogler, O.J. *Structured Mediation in Divorce Settlement.* Lexington, Massachusetts: Lexington Books, 1978.

DeBurger, James E. *Marriage Today: Problems, Issues, and Alternatives.* New York: John Wiley, 1977.

Epstein, Joseph. *Divorced in America.* New York: E.P. Dutton, 1974.

Fisher, Esther O. *Divorce: The New Freedom.* New York: Harper and Row, 1974.

Froiland, D.J. and Hozman, T.L. Counseling for constructive divorce. *Personnel and Guidance Journal*, 1977, *55*, 525-529.

Gardner, Richard A. *Psychotherapy with Children of Divorce.* New York: Jason Aronson, 1976.

Gibran, Kahlil. *The Prophet.* New York: Alfred A. Knopf, 1923.

Goode, William J. *Women in Divorce.* New York: Free Press, 1956.

Hall, Calvin S. and Lindzey, Gardner. *Theories of Personality.* (Third Edition) New York: John Wiley, 1976.

Horney, Karen. *Neuroses and Human Growth.* New York: W.W. Norton, 1950.

Hunt, Morton and Hunt, Bernice. *The Divorce Experience.* New York: McGraw-Hill, 1977.

Hyatt, I. Ralph. *Before You Marry...Again.* New York: Random House, 1977.

Johnson, Stephen M. *First Person Singular: Living the Good Life Alone.* Philadelphia: Lippincott, 1977.

Jourard, Sidney M. *Healthy Personality.* New York: Macmillan, 1974.

Jourard, Sidney. In Otto, Herbert A. and Mann, John (Eds), *Ways of Growth*. New York: Viking Press, 1962.

Kaslow, Florence W. Divorce and divorce therapy, in A. Gurman and D. Kniskern (Eds), *Handbook of Family Therapy*, New York: Brunner/Mazel, In press, 1980a.

Kaslow, Florence W. Stages of divorce: A psycholegal perspective, *Villanova Law Review*, In press, 1980b.

Kelly, J.B. and Wallerstein, J. Brief interventions with children in divorcing families. *American Journal of Orthopsychiatry*, 1977, *47*.

Kessler, Sheila. *The American Way of Divorce: Prescription for Change*. Chicago: Nelson Hall, 1975.

Kessler, Sheila and Bostwick, S. Beyond divorce: Coping skills for children. *Journal of Clinical Child Psychology*, 1977, *6*, 38-41.

Krantzler, Mel. *Creative Divorce*. New York: M. Evans, 1974.

Kubler-Ross, Elizabeth. *On Death and Dying*. New York: Macmillan, 1969.

Maslow, Abraham H. Some basic propositions of a growth and self-actualization psychology. In *Perceiving, Behaving, Becoming: A New Focus for Education*. Washington, D.C.: Yearbook of the Association for Supervision and Curriculum Development, 1962.

Rice, David. *Dual Career Marriage: Conflict and Treatment*. New York: Macmillan, 1979.

Sager, Clifford J. *Marriage Contracts and Couple Therapy*. New York: Brunner/Mazel, 1976.

Steinberg, Joseph. Toward an interdisciplinary commitment: A divorce lawyer proposes attorney-therapist marriages, or at least, an affair. *Journal of Marital and Family Therapy*, 1980, *16*, (3).

Visher, E. & Visher, J. *Stepfamilies*. New York: Brunner/Mazel, 1979.

Weiss, Robert S. *Marital Separation*. New York: Basic Books, 1975.

GRANDPARENTS OF DIVORCE
AND REMARRIAGE

Richard A. Kalish
Emily Visher

ABSTRACT. Among the individuals affected by divorce are the parents of the divorcing persons. Their role must be seen through three perspectives: that of the older persons themselves, that of the divorcing couple, and that of the children of the divorcing couple. A dozen grandparent-of-divorce settings are outlined and their implications discussed. Significant variables include which parent has custody, subsequent remarriage and the new grandparental relationships that are established, and the perceptions of the grandchildren of their new family relationships.

The role of grandparents of divorce and remarriage must be seen through at least three perspectives. First, there is the perspective of the older individuals themselves; what happens to their relationships with their children and grandchildren, how do their family involvements change, what feelings do they develop about the divorce and events

Richard A. Kalish, PhD, recently of the California School of Professional Psychology, Berkeley, is presently Clinical Professor at the Department of Psychiatry, University of New Mexico, and is a faculty member with the non-resident program of the Fielding Institute. Emily Visher, PhD, a clinical psychologist in private practice in Palo Alto, California, is a co-founder and president of Stepfamily Association of America, Inc., Palo Alto. This paper is a substantial expansion of preliminary versions presented to the Gerontological Society at their annual meeting in Washington, D.C., November 1979, and to the American Orthopsychiatric Society at their annual meeting in Toronto, April, 1980.

leading up to the divorce, what feelings do they now have concerning their own children, grandchildren, stepgrandchildren-in-law, potential or actual new children-in-law?

Second, there is the perspective of the divorcing child and child-in-law: how have they involved the older generation in their changing family structure, how have they used their parents as resources, what kinds of family tensions have developed with the parent generation, what happens as the familiar time continuum moves from separation to divorce to single parenting to new involvements to remarriage and possible stepfamilies, what happens to grandparental support or interference when remarriage occurs?

Third, inevitably, there is the perspective of the grandchildren and stepgrandchildren: how do they perceive the roles of the grandparents and stepgrandparents, what kind of relationships would they like to have and what kinds of relationships do they, in fact, have?

Given the fact that each year millions of people in the United States and Canada are newly affected by divorce, single parenting, and remarriage, it is remarkable that so little social and behavioral science data are available. Given the fact that each year marks a new role for hundreds of thousands of grandparents of divorce and remarriage, it is remarkable that virtually no demographic or other kinds of relevant data are available.

Who Are the Grandparents of Divorce and Remarriage?

Grandparents of divorce can be grandparents (or perhaps great-grandparents) who get divorced; they can be parents of people who get divorced; they can be grandparents of people who get divorced. In this article, we are primarily concerned with the middle group, those persons whose children are themselves also parents and get divorced. In the discussion that follows there are also implications for persons who are parents of single parents or who are stepgrandparents because of the marriage of their never married son or daughter to someone who has children by a prior marriage.

Unfortunately, there is, to our knowledge, no epidemiology of grandparents of divorce. We can estimate, but we do not know how many such persons there are in this country nor how many are added to the list each year. It isn't quite a matter of determining the number of divorces and multiplying by four, although we could make an estimate based on the age and social class of divorcing persons, we would still have some difficulty in determining which grandparents were newly entered into the category, grandparents of divorce, and which grandparents had been there previously, either by virtue of a previous divorce of this child or by the divorce of another child. Equally important, we don't know either the incidence or prevalance of stepgrandparenthood.

We do know that grandparents of divorce can be in their thirties or their eighties, can themselves be married, divorced, widowed, or conceivably never married, can in fact have any of the characteristics that accrue to individuals who are grandparents.

Grandparents Who Divorce

Late-life divorces are becoming increasingly common, giving rise to a relatively small, but not insignificant, group of people who have spent 20 or 40 more years as part of a married couple and now are again single, not through widowhood but through divorce. So there are adult children, 30 to 50 years of age, having to decide for the first time whether they will spend Christmas with mother's household or with father's.

The feelings of children of divorce know no age barrier. Independent sophisticated men and women often feel abandoned and betrayed, angry and depressed. Just as for a ten-year-old, the foundation of their world has cracked and their future seems unpredictable. In other instances, they are relieved and wonder why their parents took thirty years to move apart, having destroyed their own lives in a useless effort to remain together. And not infrequently, do the adult children have to absolve themselves of the responsibility for the parental marriage having lasted as long as it did, since it was "for the sake of the children" that was obviously the cement.

Grandparents Who Remarry

Grandparents also remarry, which stirs up another kind of upset and anger with their children. Resistance to a stepparent is not limited to dependent children who still live in the household; 30-year-olds and 50-year-olds may similarly resent another man sharing mother's bed or another woman sharing father's estate. Other feelings become involved, as one woman in her 50's wryly observed, "When I see my mother and her new husband snuggling up close together on the couch and looking lovingly into each other's eyes, I feel real pangs of jealousy because my own 25-year-old marriage has been feeling pretty stale and dull."

Humor often carries its own truth, and one story that has recently been making the rounds represents, like so many jokes, a basic truth. This story describes a couple in their nineties who had just applied for a divorce. They had lived together through many years of unhappiness and tension, and when asked why they had not divorced earlier, their reply was "We wanted to wait until all our children had died." Sick humor? Yes, in its way, but also instructive.

Grandparents Whose Children Divorce

The majority of grandparents of divorce, however, are grandparents whose child divorces, and the ensuing family combinations and permutations are numerous. What happens to these grandparents, to their roles and relationships, is not only a function of their own personality, health, income, and—probably most important—previous relationships with child, ex-child-in-law, and grandchildren, but also of innumerable other factors. Who has custody of the children how much of the time? Has another adult, a lover or spouse-to-be or grandparent, become involved? Are stepgrandchildren added to the mix? Or children with a subsequent spouse? How much access do these grandparents still have to their grandchildren?

With time, much of this is subject to change. The grandchild who cannot spend enough time with Grandma at three or seven may have deeply involving social relationships at 13 or 17; the grandparent who is working fulltime when the divorce first occurs may retire and have much more available time three years later.

There follows in outline form a dozen grandparent-of-divorce settings. These are far from inclusive, but they may help raise consciousness about the complexities of the grandparent-of-divorce and remarriage role.

When the Adult Child Retains Custody

First, there are grandparents whose divorced child retains custody of the children. These grandparents may be re-enlisted as baby-sitters, advice-givers, financial-supporters, in all ways that they had been pulling back from (or pushed away from) during the previous year. Households may merge, perhaps two grandparents, one parent, and one or more children, since it is easier to divide money and childcare roles than for the single parent to operate alone with the children. There is a price to pay, of course, in loss of privacy and of autonomy, in providing grand-parents with responsibilities that they had believed were shed some years earlier, and in physical crowding, but it may be worth the price.

Often these grandparents become close to the grandchildren and play a semi-parental role, whether they share in the household or reside separately. The grandfather may become the most signficant man in the lives of the young children; the grandmother may supplant the mother if the latter's work and social demands become sufficiently absorbing. (Many of the concerns of divorced parents resemble the concerns of families where both parents are employed outside of the home on a fulltime basis.)

Second, there are grandparents whose divorced child retains custody of the children, and then remarries a person who has no children. Now the grandparents may have some competition, and if they have acted in a semi-parental role and have formed close bonds with their grand-children, their sense of loss, and at times their anger from this loss, can be profound. It may have been stressful for them when their child first married, and more stressful when the divorce occurred, but they survived both by adapting effectively. Now they confront another change in their child's family status, accompanied by the knowledge that not only is their child vulnerable to the problems of a marriage but that their grand-children are even more vulnerable to someone who may not even love them "like a parent should."

On the other hand, grandparents are often relieved when the remar-riage occurs, since they experience an unexpected return to greater intimacy away from the substantial expenditure of time and energy (and sometimes money) on their grandchildren that can be taken over by the new spouse. The older people may feel now they can return to a life of minimal family responsibilities. Although research is lacking, we surmise that the anxieties of grandparents tend to continue nevertheless. Grand-parents are likely to be tense, especially early in the remarriage: how will he treat *my* grandchildren? Will she persuade him to move away? Am I going to be able to keep my key to the house?

Third, there are grandparents whose child is divorced and retains custody of the grandchildren, who remarries a person who has children, although the children are not going to reside regularly in the re-formed household. Perhaps the children are old enough to be living on their own, perhaps they are residing with the former spouse of the new child-in-law, perhaps they are at boarding school or living with another set of grand-parents or rooming with a friend and that person's family.

Whatever the situation, the grandparents also become stepgrandparents. How do they treat these new stepgrandchildren? If they buy their own grandchild a ten-speed bicycle for Christmas, can they get away with a 1000-piece picture puzzle for their stepgrandchild? If they take their own grandchild to Disneyland, must their stepgrandchild accompany them? Does it matter if the stepgrandchildren have their own grandparents or not?

You do not have to love or even like your own grandchildren, but you almost always do. You do not have to love or even like your new stepgrandchildren, and although you would like to love them and certainly to like them, you can not always do so. Grandparents, like parents and children, develop a family system, and intruders may never be fully integrated into that system. Grandparents view new stepgrandchildren with much the same eyes as parents view new stepchildren, except that the latter at least chose the relationship that led to the children, even if they didn't choose the children. Stepgrandparents, on the other hand, selected neither the relationship nor the children and may very well be displeased with both. This is not the place to discuss the stresses of stepparenting, but it does seem appropriate to point out that most of the difficulties encountered by stepparents are also encountered by stepgrandparents, although usually at a diminished level of intensity (see Lofas & Roosevelt, 1976, and Visher & Visher, 1979, for futher discussion of stepfamilies).

To some extent, the tension is reduced for these grandparents because they can visit their own grandchildren without having to deal with their stepgrandchildren at the same time. Gifts may not be compared when the two sets of children live in different households. Actual personal contacts are infrequent, and their grandchildren are seldom required to share their toys, clothes, or parents with the new stepsiblings because of living in separate households.

Fourth, there are grandparents whose child is divorced and retains custody of the grandchildren, who remarries a person with children who do reside regularly in the re-formed household. Now everything outlined above applies *and* the stepgrandchildren are there also, virtually all of the time. The old coziness of grandparents, parents, and grandchildren together is no more. The older people not only have to deal with a new marriage and new spouse for their child, but they have to deal with one or two or three or more other unfamiliar people in the household. Now their beloved grandchildren are being bossed around by unwanted older stepsiblings or being annoyed by unwanted younger stepsiblings; bedrooms are now being shared; toys and clothes become interchangeable.

It takes time for new relationships to develop, even though these stepsibling relationships have usually developed some history prior to the marriage. If the relationships between the children work out well, the grandparents may look more favorably on their new stepkin; if competition and tension develop between the two sets of children, the grandparents are likely to take sides and they may bring pressure on their own child to take a similar position.

Gift-giving can become a time of major trial and tribulation. On their modest incomes (or while saving for retirement), the grandparents didn't mind scrimping a bit to get these two grandchildren nice presents for birthdays and Christmas. Now there are three more youngsters to deal with, and they must either spend considerably more money, reduce substantially the amount spent for their own grandchildren, or do some of each.

A fifth setting, one that occurs frequently, may have no particular effect on the grandparents: a new infant being born into the remarriage. Since the grandparents are just as much grandparents of this new infant as of the other children, they may be pleased with its arrival. Only if their relationship with their new child-in-law is unhappy, is the new baby likely to add difficulty. (This, of course, ignores all the other reasons that they might be making them unhappy, but such reasons are not related to the divorce-remarriage situation.)

When the Divorced Adult Child Does Not Retain Custody

Another set of situations develop when the divorced child of these grandparents does not retain physical custody of the children. Such grandparents frequently have great difficulty in maintaining a relationship with their grandchildren, because no legal tie remains between them and their child's former spouse. During the divorce, the older persons normally support the position of their own child. After the dust settles, they may be isolated from their former child-in-law and, therefore, from their grandchildren. The courts set up the rights of the non-custodial parent, but the courts rarely if ever provide the grandparents of divorce with visitation rights. (Although a newspaper article in early 1980 did report an instance when this occurred, based in large part on the continued involvement and financial support provided by the grandparents.)

If the father (or the mother, if she is the non-custodial parent) does not maintain contact with the children or provide the child support, the former daughter-in-law may make it difficult or impossible for the father to see the children, and she is likely to treat his parents in the same fashion. Even if the non-custodial parent does have ready access to his children, his former spouse does not have to accommodate his parents. This can mean that the grandparents are able only to be with their grandchildren at those times that their son (or daughter) can be with them. Although the grandparents may have invested heavily of themselves, of their affect and their energies, in their grandchildren, they can find their access cut off or, at the very least, greatly limited. And even if this does not occur, grandparents often fear that it might occur.

The sixth situation just described faces the grandparents whose child is divorced and whose grandchildren are living with their former child-in-law who remains single. If the former child-in-law is remarried, or perhaps living with someone, the circumstances become still more stressful. In this seventh situation, the older couple has to recognize that their grandchildren, their flesh and blood, their heirs, their descendents, are living with *two* people to whom the grandparents themselves are no longer related. One of these two people may still be angry because of the events surrounding the divorce, and the other is someone the grandparents do not even know, who may care nothing for their grandchildren, and who has only modest obligations to the youngsters and none to the grandparents.

The next three settings closely resemble the seventh setting, discussed above. These are eighth, the grandparents whose child is divorced and whose grandchildren are living with their former child-in-law who has remarried someone with children not in the household; ninth, grandparents whose child is divorced and whose grandchildren are living with their former child-in-law who is remarried to someone with children residing in the household; tenth, grandparents whose child is divorced and whose grandchildren are living with their former child-in-law who is remarried and has a subsequent infant in this marriage.

Eleventh, there are grandparents whose child is divorced, remarried and re-divorced. If these grandparents have developed any kind of positive relationship with their stepgrandchildren, it may be destroyed by the re-divorce. If, of course, they had developed stressful relationships with the stepgrandchildren, the re-divorce can reduce the tension, and now the grandparents may re-engage with their own grandchildren more fully.

The twelfth condition does alter our original definition somewhat, but still seems to deserve recognition. In some instances, stepgrandparenthood is conferred upon people who had not been grandparents, at least with that particular child, previously. These people do not have bloodline grandchildren involved in the marriage or re-marriage, although their sudden new role may either elicit or destroy certain long-cherished fantasies about becoming grandparents. In one instance, a man in his early twenties married a divorced 34-year-old woman with three children. It is unlikely that his parents, barely a decade older than their daughter-in-law had previously anticipated being quickly thrust into the stepgrandparenthood of three boys ranging in age from 9 to 13.

The related situation, when someone who has never had children and is nearing the outer limits of safe parenting age becomes a stepparent through marriage, has a more variable effect on the newly ordained stepgrandparents. They might be greatly pleased to be offered the opportunity they had probably felt they had missed, or they may be less than pleased at the turn of events.

There are also grandparents whose divorced child is living with someone without legal marriage, or whose divorced child is now part of a homosexual couple, or whose divorced child has adopted the children of his former wife's previous marriage, and so on ad infinitum. The recoupling patterns of divorce-marriage chains confronting grandparents of divorce seem infinite in number.

Some Implications

Like everyone else in the family system, the participation of grandparents of divorce and remarriage can improve the well-being of other members or detract from that well-being or, most likely, do some of each. Changes are difficult, particularly changes over which the individual has little or no control. Grandparents of divorce and remarriage are faced with caring for a family tree bearing strange and unfamiliar fruit; the tree no longer resembles the tree they have known and nurtured, and they may be faced with conflicting emotions and difficult choices.

Also like others in the family system, the choices these grandparents make will affect the entire system. In fact, they can be instrumental in the success or failure of their child's single parenting, post-divorce life, and eventual remarriage. Like the children of the newly married couple, grandparents are capable of putting a wedge between the husband and wife.

Agnes, a 36-year-old mother of three children, had been remarried to Frank for three years. Frank had been a fairly successful stepfather, although not without some tensions developed from his guilt about not spending enough time with his own children from his former marriage, who lived with their mother. Christmas had been routinely spent by everyone at Frank's parents' home, but this year Agnes' children absolutely refused to go.

At first they wouldn't explain, perhaps fearing that their reasons would not be adequate, but eventually they told Agnes that they always received token gifts from their stepgrandparents, while their stepbrothers and stepsister had been getting major gifts. To make matters worse, the size of the gift was mirrored in the ways they were treated by their stepgrandparents. It wasn't that the older people were cruel, but that they weren't interested in these children, and made only minimal pretense that they were interested.

The older couple saw themselves as being nice to everyone, but did not feel it necessary to treat all children equally. Their son saw the scene from the same position, especially since he was, in his own eyes, helping support his wife's children from her previous marriage. Agnes realized her children were not treated as equals, but felt she was not entitled to make demands on either her husband or her mother-in-law, since the child support she received did not cover all expenses that her children incurred. And her children only saw themselves as being ignored, as being excluded from the conversations, as getting token gifts; they had gotten together and decided to stop going.

In effect, grandparents find in divorce an entirely new set of circumstances, roles for which our society prescribes behavior only in the most fuzzy fashion. These persons have their own fears and anxieties; they're often isolated from grandchildren they love; they are no longer secure that their inheritance will reach the people they wish it to reach; they sometimes watch youngsters they love deeply being reared by people for whom they have no regard and with whom they are likely to have no influence. So when we speak about the powerlessness of older people, few roles have less power than grandparents whose divorced child does not have custody of the grandchildren, and where the relationships between adults involved with the grandchildren are less than cordial.

In many instances, however, grandparents do have power and can be important in what happens. Unfortunately, their power is often directed against the potential for a good new relationship that their divorced child may be trying to create. The grandparents may build walls in a remarriage setting rather than building bridges. And in a remarriage, dependent children have particular difficulty with conflicting feelings about the new adults in their lives, so that the support or undermining by grandparents can be a highly significant factor.

Although a child may find it strange to have a new father or mother, having a new grandfather or grandmother does not seem strange—they've always had a couple of them anyway. Therefore, if stepgrandparents include these children in their lives, the children may come to see their new stepparent as responsible for bringing something valuable to them. After all, the pleasure of a trip to the zoo with the parents of a new stepfather can lead the children to consider that the man their mother married has offered them something more than orders to keep their rooms clean and their stereo turned down.

Stress-Producing Patterns

There appear to be six major patterns involving grandparents of divorce and remarriage that create difficulties.

The first centers on the new couple and their relationship. Often a stepfamily has worked through its initial problems and is functioning reasonably smoothly when the grandparents arrive on the scene and point out to their remarried child that the new spouse is not treating their grandchild in a sufficiently loving and thoughtful manner. Suddenly the remarried parent sees the stepparent-stepchild relationship through new eyes.

Paul had felt guilty about the pain his divorce had caused his children, and he had worked hard to make it up to them. Sally, his new wife, had not been married before and did not especially want to have children of her own, but she was pleased with the opportunity of being a stepmother to 8-year-old Julie who was always so charming. She under-estimated the strength of the system that Julie and Paul had built during their four years together, and she didn't realize how Julie would pull her in-laws into the game.

Whenever Sally attempted to discipline Julie with the grandparents around, the child looked to them for support, increasing Sally's tension level many fold. Eventually Paul was told by his parents that Julie was being verbally abused by Sally, and Paul's own perception of the situation, influenced by Sally's greater tension, essentially confirmed his parents' observations. Paul asked Sally to "get off Julie's back," which led to an argument that was to wax and wane for several weeks. And whenever things became a little more relaxed, Paul's parents would return to pressure him with more disapproving glances.

In another case, a totally different dynamic occurred. Here the new wife had read in a magazine about the possible damage that grandparents can cause, and she worked diligently to create a new family system that would keep her future mother-in-law away, although not so far away that the older woman would be denied access to the children. However, both the husband and his children were confused by the new structure, and the older woman, deeply hurt and confused, withdrew from the family. The result was angry arguments between husband and wife that were never fully reconciled.

The second pattern centers on the remarried adult child who feels caught between his or her parents, children, and, perhaps, ex-spouse on one side and his or her stepchildren and present spouse on the other side. The usual pattern of complaints from his former wife that his child support payments do not cover her costs vie with complaints from his present wife that he is giving more money in child support than he needs to. When his parents enter the fray, the tension mounts, as conflicting loyalties seem tied to irreconcilable choices. In such a situation, the remarried child may withdraw and become alienated and alone, pulled by competing sets of people and wanting to separate them from each other.

Third, in extreme cases, grandparents may actively seek to break up their child's new marriage, and they may recruit their grandchildren as allies in their struggle. This places the grandchildren between the grandparents whom they love and their parent whom they also love, perhaps in tandem with their stepparent whom they may or may not care for. This is much like the previous pattern, except the young children are caught in the middle of an intergenerational battle instead of a battle between spouses or ex-spouses.

Tony couldn't understand why his 11-year-old daughter, Louise, always returned tense, demanding, even hysterical from visits to his parents. On one occasion, she shrieked at him that he had been ''so awful to Grandma and Grandpa that I hate you.'' Tony's new wife, Polly, figured out that the grandparents had grown to enjoy their revived parenting role after the divorce, and they felt that Polly had married Tony primarily to have a father for her children, which they resented. As a result, they continued to remind Polly's stepdaughter, Louise, of how much nicer her life had been before she had to share a bedroom with her step-sister and when ''Grandma cooked dinner for you almost every night instead of that woman who works all day and is too tired to cook a really good meal.''

At times, the grandparents even mentioned that they could all be together again, if Tony were only to divorce Polly. Louise, caught in this terrible crossfire, including innuendo that Tony no longer cared for his parents, feeling divided because of her love for her father and his well-being and her love for her grandparents, became increasingly tense and eventually hysterical.

At this point, Tony and Polly sought professional help, and Tony realized that he had permitted the conflict to get out of hand. A session with both the younger couple and the older couple, who in spite of their anger wanted their son and granddaughter to be happy, provided the adults with enough insight into what they were doing to the young girl to get them to leave Louise outside of the conflict arena.

A fourth troublesome pattern emerges when the new stepparent and stepgrandchildren are not acknowledged by the new parents-in-law/step-grandparents. Time frequently mellows the emotional climate, but unfortunately even 10 or 12 years of remarriage is not always enough to enable stepgrandparents to admit that the marriage has occurred. One woman with two children had been remarried for nearly 10 years when her brother's wedding was announced. She and her children received invitations to attend, but there was no mention or any form of implicit inclusion of her husband of 10 years or of her stepchildren, who had lived with them for eight years.

The fifth complication concerns money and inheritance. In step-families where both wife and husband come from similar, preferably financially modest, backgrounds, this may not be a problem. But grandparents who can relate reasonably well to both grandchildren and step-grandchildren may give way to virtual fury at the thought that their financial assets might be divided among grandchildren and stepgrand-children. Often the remarried child is sensitive to the emotional meaning of special heirlooms, perhaps great-grandmother's diamond ring or a Seventeenth Century diningroom set, and provisions are made for such items to remain in the line of direct descent.

At the same time, unequal divisions of money or other material goods can engender strong emotional response. Her children's grandparents have promised each child a car for graduation and have provided a trust fund to cover all college expenses; his children have only the support available through him. She and her children feel that too much of their present family's money is going to subsidize his children; he and his children feel that her children have tremendous advantages in getting started in adult life that aren't available to them. And many of these circumstances will occur, even if the grandparents have died, since wills and trust funds can produce a continuing reminder of past stresses.

The sixth remarriage pattern that poses problems involving grandparents is the stepfamily with ''his,'' ''hers,'' and then ''ours.'' Suddenly the older people have a grandchild in the new family unit that ties them to the new spouse of their remarried child. Although this often helps bring the family together, it can establish its own difficult tension, especially if the new child receives so much attention that the older children and stepchildren alike are shunted into the background. Since the new child is the only one that has two parents in the family, the older children may feel more threatened and abandoned than after the birth of a brother or sister in the more familiar biological family. Grandparents, like parents, are likely to ignore the older children as they attend to the family's newest member.

Divorce and remarriage bring unanticipated upheaval and uncertainty to grandparents, causing a kaleidoscope of emotions. Many grandparents are sensitive to the interplay of emotions and work very hard to move with the changing patterns, often asking their divorced and remarried children for guidelines of acceptable behavior. In these and in many other situations, very helpful and meaningful relationships develop among the three generations, to the enrichment of all. Grandparents may have favorites in any type of family, but many become acutely sensitive to importance of equality among the children, even though this often ''feels unnatural'', especially at first. All the children get a trip to the beach, all receive presents of equal significance on their birthdays, all know that their feelings are valued. This helps produce family harmony and a warm glow in all directions.

If divorced and remarried children will offer their children's grandparents warm relationship possibilities, even if the grandparents are parents of the former spouse, these older persons will have the opportunity to become very special people in the lives of their grandchildren and stepgrandchildren. It is difficult to love again, after being hurt, but many grandparents of divorce and remarriage have been able to build bridges rather than walls, and they find the rewards well worth the risks involved.

REFERENCES

Roosevelt, Ruth & Lofas, Jeannette. *Living in step.* New York: Stein & Day, 1976.
Visher, Emily B. & Visher, John S. *Stepfamilies: A guide to working with stepparents and stepchildren.* New York: Brunner/Mazel, 1979.

CAN FAMILY RELATIONSHIPS BE MAINTAINED AFTER DIVORCE?

Janice Goldman

ABSTRACT. In this paper, the current functioning of extended families is described, as well as how that functioning is altered at the family level by the adjustment required when separation and divorce occur. A case study of a large and functional Jewish family is presented in order to explore changes in membership inclusion after divorce. A majority of family respondents still include divorced/separated affines, although not as highly as intermarried, a contrasting group. Relationships after divorce tend to be reciprocally negotiated, and subject to election based on the degree of positive regard for a former affine. Finally, this study may reflect a picture of the time interval just after separation and/or divorce, which may be essentially altered by the further passage of time and/or the remarriage status of former affines.

Notes on the Functions of Extended Families

This paper seeks to examine the nature of family relationships in the larger extended family, how its individual members relate to each other and function individually and as a family group first, in relation to nuclear families, and second in terms of social change and the specific effects wrought by separation and divorce on extended family membership. It will inquire into the mutual articulation of relationships following separation and divorce by way of a case study of a large, functional extended family which tends toward being an open system in its member-

Janice Goldman, Psy.D., is affiliated with Hahnemann Medical College & Hospital, Philadelphia, PA 19102.

ship definition. The method used included a questionnaire and the development of a genogram and family history. The purpose of this work was to aid in suggesting emergent trends to be used to define relationships in the broader context of the extended family following separation and divorce.

What is the ideal relationship between nuclear and extended families? As one respondent to the questionnaire reported: "Mainly I derive emotional satisfaction or pleasure of some sort from each close tie which I feel toward an extended family member. It is the same feeling of belonging and sharing which one feels toward one's immediate family, I suppose, except that this serves to increase or 'extend' that feeling."

Because of this feeling that members of the nuclear family derive from the broader extended family, the nuclear family continues to exist, in varying degrees, under the protective umbrella of the extended family. The kin network links many nuclear families and acts to extend functionally the workings of the immediate family, especially in times of stress. In events of crisis such as illness, accident or death, in financial hardship and old age the kin network is activated and provides its members with support and needed services.

For much of human history kinship bonds have constituted a court of last resort for the individual when his or her immediate family's coping resources were exhausted. Virtually every family, for example, has its stories of collections taken up for food and housing, and of relatives who moved in with more fortunate family members during the Great Depression. In the more affluent times since World War II in this country, families have tended to drift apart as they have less drastic need of each other. Ties of affinity have replaced the bonds of kinship, at least for the middle class. Choices of how time is invested are made based on friendship rather than on blood.

Similarly, social agencies have replaced the services once rendered by the extended family. We now see day care centers doing what grandmothers or aunts once did to ease the burdens of young mothers, while professional counselors have taken over the advice-giving functions once assumed by family elders. Friends may as often be approached for help as family members in youth through mid-life. In old age with its vicissitudes of health and financial hardship, the kin structure seems again to be called on, and if functional, will again sustain its members.

One function which appears to remain central to the extended family is the acknowledgement of the individual's passage through the life cycle. Milestone life events are important in this regard, and a major kin function seems to lie in the wider social acknowledgment of the taking on of new roles and changes in status through attendance at rites of passage. Indeed the importance of this function is attested to by the degree of hurt feelings and breaches in family relationships that occur when this function is abrogated or aborted by either party.

These larger functions then, are supported through the maintenance of relationships at different system levels, which principally occur through visitation and communication. Various investigators have found that neither geographical closeness nor hierarchical authority is necessary to sustain such extended family relationships (Litwak, 1960). Further, in spite of geographical dispersion, the use of the telephone mitigates against diminshed contact (Leitcher and Mitchell, 1968). Leitcher and Mitchell also found that failure to communicate by phone with relatives was viewed as a breach of kinship obligations as much as any other failure to interact.

Talcott Parsons (1943) detailed the kinship structure of the United States and described the American system as a conjugal one made up exclusively of interlocking conjugal families. The principle underlying the structural relation of families is that in the "structurally normal" case, the individual is a member (and the only member) of not one but two conjugal families. These are called the family of orientation and the family of procreation. The isolated conjugal family is considered the normal family unit whose members pool their resources to form a base of common support. The immediate consequence of this lies in the structural importance it imparts to the marital relationship as the keystone of the kinship system (Parsons, 1943).

In a contrasting view, Uzoka (1979) saw the modern emphasis on the nuclear family as a myth which has been propagated by western society to deal with the anguish of separation from the family necessitated by the demands of industrialization. He asserts that "the extended family is real in human terms, and that in a psychological sense, it was always there albeit invisible". He further suggests that the nuclear mythology generates unneeded anguish and loneliness in overlooking kinship supports (Uzoka, 1979). Uzoka concurs with Sussman and Burchinal (1962) who add their perception that family patterns of mutual aid are organized into what they term a 'modified extended family' adapted to contemporary urban and industrial society. Their view is that the modified extended family functions indirectly rather than directly to facilitate the achievement of both component families and individual members. Its major activities lie in mutual aid and social activity among kin related families.

Its role in relation to the nuclear family is supportive rather than coercive (Sussman and Burchinal, 1962).

At this juncture we may well ask what the extended family is in an existential sense? And where is its locus? The extended family would seem to exist as a set of potentials to be activated in times of ritual and of celebration, in times of crisis and of changes in membership. Its members define themselves and participate in shared definitions of others. As an unseen structure of affection and shared obligation, it provides the undergirding of individual lives. It exists preeminently in the minds of its members and is called into being selectively at relevant times; and only sometimes does it take on full physical form. Traditionally one enters through birth or marriage and exits only through death. In recent times divorce and separation have added a new parameter to this traditional definition.

How does separation or divorce from a family member change one's membership in the extended family? How is this transaction perceived by the divorced one and how by the family? What rules then govern what happens in the interactions between them? These questions take on special significance in this time of ''epidemic'' divorce and widespread dissolution of family bonds.

It is interesting that little has been written to date that directly addresses the description of kinship interaction after divorce. Spicer and Hampe (1975) have found that affectional and obligational bonds with affines is weakened or eliminated following divorce while bonds with the consanguineous family remained stable or increased, as measured by frequency of contact. There was a tendency for females to have more frequent contact than males with both consanguines and affines after divorce, and this was particularly influenced by the presence of children for females. The rate of contact of the male and female divorcee was seen to decrease as one progressed outward from the nuclear family for both consanguines and former affines. These findings were seen to document the central position of the female in the kin structure, especially as a mother of children, which pushes the female toward kin contact. Spicer and Hampe (1975) go on to suggest that the presence of children is crucial, creating a feeling on the part of the divorcee that the children are connected to the former affines by a blood relationship. In itself this perception creates a feeling of obligation to continue the interaction. They add that being female, the presence of children becomes a functional equivalent for the marital bond in maintaining contact after a divorce with affinal relatives (Spicer and Hampe, 1975).

A Case Study of Divorce in An Extended Family

The following is a case study of the impact of divorce in a large functional extended family covering four generations. The purpose is to see how in this one family, family relationships continued to be maintained after divorce. To understand its functional patterns, it is important to look first to the history of the family and of its founding matriarch and patriarch. A genogram will be presented and then the questionnaire data will follow. In this description it becomes important to note the special characteristics of Jewish extended families. Leitcher and Mitchell (1968) have reported that Jewish kin networks are large and tend to extend laterally with less generational depth and fluid outer boundaries. Some degree of interaction tends to be maintained with a high proportion of recognized living kin. Geographical proximity to kin is valued and is supported behaviorally. Emotional ties are reinforced by acts of instrumental assistance, and Jewish families are involved in the reciprocity of give and take. Thus, Jewish families, as a distinct ethnic group, tend to be deeply involved with their kin (Leitcher and Mitchell, 1968).

The G. Family

Historical data of the G. family is available from 1894 when two Jewish immigrants from Russia, both from the vicinity of Kiev, were married. Both immigrated to the United States as adolescents. Mother stayed at the home of relatives and Father was a boarder there and so they met. They did not know each other prior to their meeting. By 1894 they were married and they had the first of their eight children by 1895.

Father began as a huckster with a pack on his back. He sold soft disposables and rags and this evolved to a horse and wagon business and finally to the founding of a paper stock company. As the paper business became successful, he turned it over to his second son, his brother and his brother-in-law. Then as money was accumulated he invested in mortgages and real estate, and became a wealthy man by the standards of his time. Much of this wealth was in the leverage real estate of that day which crumbled in the Great Depression. Father lay on his deathbed in the early

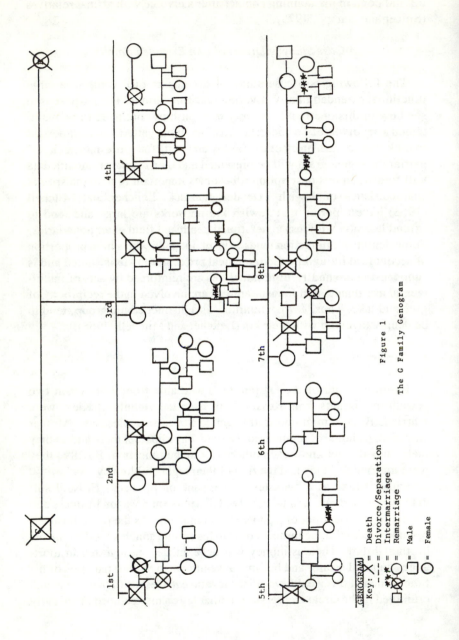

Figure 1

The G Family Genogram

GENOGRAM
Key: X = Death
     - - - = Divorce/Separation
     ∗∗∗ = Intermarriage
     ⊗ = Remarriage
     □ = Male
     ○ = Female

1930s as his four sons met to salvage what they could of the family fortunes.

Father is remembered as a strict, very severe man, who was held in the highest respect by his children. He loved his family and was a strict constructionist of family boundaries. For example, a story is told of a family trip to a nearby seaside resort where the family stopped for lunch in a roadside restaurant. At this time, some of the children were married, and one of his daughters-in-law took a seat next to Father. Father exploded and pushed her away, saying he wanted one of his *own* children next to him.

Yet Father was adaptive in relation to the American culture and was the first to own many of the new technological gadgets: the first telephone, the first crystal set, the first of many new automobiles was his. After World War I, for instance, he went to see the new airplanes for himself and took a ride with each of his children when considering whether to invest in surplus planes. He even advertised in the newspapers for people with inventions to come to his house so that he could see whether he wished to back them financially. He was stricter with his daughters than with his sons and ordered them about even after they had married. On the other hand, he sometimes relented and moved toward the ways of the new country where his children were concerned. For example, he joined a conservative synagogue so that his younger two daughters might receive a religious education which was not available to women in the strict orthodox tradition.

Mother, in contrast, was remembered as a warmer and softer person, the fairest woman to all of her children. She mediated for them with father and acted as a go-between in family dissension, smoothing over the rough places. She was charitable and worked in the synagogue and for philanthropic causes before the days of organized charity. There was domestic help in the house, and mother, in advance of her time, went to the real estate office to work alongside of father until one or another family emergency might pull her back. However, through a part of his business life she was not readily included by father in his pleasures. When he went to the opera he loved or to the movies, he was more apt to take along one of the children.

Everyone loved Mother as they respected Father. She was warm, outgoing, and embraced everyone, the people her children married as well as her children. She too adapted to American ways, and her adaptation was more in the personal than the cultural realm. For instance, she herself kept a kosher house, but she visited each of her married children and gave them permission to decide for themselves whether they wished to keep kosher.

Thus, there were two forces in the family embodied in its founding parents; a force of strict construction promoting unity and a strong boundary of family membership, and a force promoting a "soft" definition and geared to family adaptation. These forces in combination were to provide for the life of this family and its health over the next four generations as its members prospered and grew in number.

Eight children were born to the family, four sons and four daughters in alternating pairs, spaced roughly every two years. All the sons were given Americanized English names, while the daughters were given the traditional names of Yiddish culture. It was as if a split adaptational message was bestowed from the first, namely that the sons were to adapt to the new land and go out from the family while the daughters were to remain close and uphold the traditional family norms. Thus was the pace of family adaptation to be monitored to satisfy two contradictory wishes: the wish to change and assimilate, and the wish to remain with the familiar and the known. This was further underscored by offering each of the sons but not the older two of the four daughters a college education. By the time of the younger daughters' graduation from high school, Father and family had relented somewhat and these women went on to higher education.

The G. family continued in the second generation to be close, stable and to prosper as a family and as individuals. Dysfunction was concentrated in one of eight children and in his progeny, leaving other family members relatively free. Dysfunction and stress also tended to be expressed and experienced physiologically rather than psychologically or socially. Heart disease was widespread through the eight siblings and none of the males survived it beyond the age of 69. The women, now in their mid to late seventies and early eighties are also touched by heart disease, although all four are surviving.

Divorce has come later to this clan than to the general population. Only in the last five years have two separations/divorces occurred in the third generation in marriages of fifteen years plus duration. There was one earlier divorce in the fourth generation of a less than two year marriage in the sibling line where familial dysfunction was concentrated. The clan, which spans four living generations now numbers some eighty-two to eighty-four living members. It still continues to meet regularly for two yearly events to which all members are invited: a family seder and a family picnic.

This family continues to be functional. There are few emotional cut-offs of members and inclusion is high. When a member of the family dies and his or her spouse remarries, the new couple continue to be regarded as family members. There are two physicians who offer medical service without charge, and legal or business advice is also frequently exchanged. Direct financial aid is offered currently to one member of the second generation. Emotional support and individual feelings of belonging are widespread among the second and third generation, but may be waning in the fourth. There are many friendships and elective social interactions.

G. Family's Reactions to Divorce Among Its Members

It is of interest to see how such a favored family regards separation and divorce. With its high rate of inclusion, are separated and divorced spouses still to be regarded as family members? To answer this question, a questionnaire was distributed at a family event to all adult family members present and mailed to a random sample of those not present. Forty-five questionnaires in all were distributed to members of three generations. Thirteen eligible members did not receive questionnaires.

The rate of return of questionnaires overall was some 40%. Out of the second generation with ten living family members, there was a 70% return. In the third generation out of a possible twenty-three members (one disqualified) 56% were returned. In the fourth generation with twenty-four members over the age of 21, only three questionnaires were returned, making the response rate here only 12%. Perhaps this is a commentary in itself on the future of the family, although in the family as presently constituted feelings of commitment run high.

Inclusion of a separated or divorced spouse was touched on in two ways. Family members were asked to list in various ways who was in the family and which family members would be invited to a given event if they were hosting. The family picnic which traditionally includes all family members regardless of age is an example of a family event which rotates among third generation family members, who electively take responsibility for organizing it and issuing invitations. Family members were also asked to share their direct perception of whether a divorced or separated member was still to be considered part of the family once they were divorced or separated from the "blood" relatives. The same questions were asked in relation to the issue of intermarriage as a control, as whether intermarried members, i.e., non-Jews, were considered full and included family members. In the first and second generations, marriage within the Jewish religion was total and in Father's will, all grandchildren who might marry a non-Jew were to be disinherited totally. The issue of intermarriage had arisen, and was prohibited with economic sanction.

Results of the questionnaire are tabulated in Tables 1 to 4 as follows.

Discussion of Results

Table 1 which tabulates the responses to questions touching on the inclusion of separated and divorced affinial family members measured by invitation to events shows some interesting trends. The older generation is split in their perception as to whether such persons would be included; twice as many people in the middle generation would tend to include as to exclude, and the youngest generation does not see this question as pertaining to themselves. Similar patterns prevail in the question touching internal perceptions of membership (Table 2). Of special interest is the response category labeled Qualified. Here respondents demarcated the interactional nature of negotiating continuing relationships following separation and divorce by such statements as "it would be up to them," and "if a relationship existed between me and a divorced cousin...it would not sever a friendship." Respondents stressed that to remain in the extended family the divorced or separated one would have to make an effort to communicate or have some relationship to counter the drift away.

Table 3 reports percentages of membership inclusion over the three adult generations queried. It provides a comparison with the intermarriage and its effect on status of inclusion. It can be seen that intermarried family members enjoy a higher rate of inclusion than do divorced or separated members. Although the difference between 64% combined full and qualified inclusion for intermarried members and 52% inclusion for divorced/separated members does not in itself seem significant, the no inclusion category for both groups contains a telling comparison. *No* intermarried member is excluded either behaviorally or perceptually, while 34% of family members would not continue to include divorced or separated members. The no response category for intermarriage is also quite high at 36%, indicating perhaps that intermarriage is not considered an issue worthy of much fuss one way or the other.

Another interesting trend not reflected in the tables is contained in the qualitative aspect of responses; namely, the mention of liking or dislik-

Table 1.

Inclusion of a Separated or Divorced Member as Measured
by Invitation to Events

	Yes, Would Include	No, Excluded	Other or Qualified	Total
Second Generation (7 respondents)	3	3	1	7
Third Generation (13 respondents)	6	3	4	13
Fourth Generation (3 respondents)	0	0	3*	3

*Young adult members of the fourth generation have not yet hosted such events and do not see themselves as so doing.

Table 2.

Inclusion of a Separated or Divorced Person in Perception
as Still Being Part of Family by Generation

	Yes	No	Qualified	Total
Second Generation	3	3	1	7
Third Generation	5	3	5	13
Fourth Generation	0	2	1	3

Table 3.

Comparison of Separated/Divorced and Intermarried Family Members
as to Status of Inclusion (Events and Perceptions Combined) by
Percentage of Respondents

	Full Inclusion	Qualified Inclusion	No Inclusion	Non-Scorable Response	Total
Separated/Divorced	26%	26%	34%	14%	100%
	(52%)				
Intermarried	60%	4%	0%	36%	100%
	(64%)				

153

Table 4.

Comparison of Separated/Divorced and Intermarried Family Members
as to Status of Inclusion (Events and Perceptions Combined) by
Percentage of Respondents

	Full Inclusion	Qualified Inclusion		No Inclusion	Non-Scorable Response	Total
Separated/Divorced	26%	26%	(52%)	34%	14%	100%
Intermarried	60%	4%	(64%)	0%	36%	100%

ing a given family member as a rationale for continuing relationships beyond the definitional inclusion as family. Such a position is reflected in the following quote:

> My feelings for the divorced G. cousins haven't changed at all. My regard for the other spouse is a function of my feelings toward them as individuals, considerations of membership aside—if I liked them before, I continue to like them, (i.e., regard them as family); if I didn't like them, I'd prefer breaking the tie.

Perhaps this kind of response, which was found in both second and third generational respondents, is reflective of the movement noted previously to the replacement of family ties with friendship ties. A blending of friend and family occurs as an intermediate category and takes on elective properties to be decided by the individual.

A view from the other side is provided by the divorced or separated members all of whom are women: two are former affines and one a G. consanguine who provides a perspective on a different family group. All three have children and mention the motivation to keep extended family ties for the sake of the children. Again the interactional and negotiated aspect of family relationships after separation and divorce is paramount. Business ties and services exchanged tend to continue more easily than face-to-face social interaction. Attendance at events after an invitation is offered is dependent on whether the former spouse (who has first choice) will be present. The discomfort which would be projected and felt were the former mate to be present with a new female, mitigates against full attendance. Both former affines of the G. family, however, stress their perception of feeling included and still welcomed. The maintenance of specific relationships, as before, tend to follow friendship lines.

In contrast, the G. consanguine had a different experience where she was refused in spite of her efforts to maintain relationships. She notes that when first separated she had a "fairly decent relationship" with her husband's family, but somehow it began to deteriorate through the years. She attributes this to deaths and remarriage in the immediate family and to external problems. She writes "The efforts I made were mostly on (my child's) behalf, but I stopped trying when my efforts were not reciprocated." To the question "Does any life event change a person's membership in the family?" she writes, "Theoretically, it should not. The difference would arise from how comfortable other family members feel with intermarriage or divorce, such as what situation caused the divorce."

Additionally, both former affines in the G. family note that attendance at events and membership status will be changed should they remarry. At such a juncture, they project that the choice would be to either come alone to family events or to sever ties with the extended family. Thus the present picture described may reflect a transitional time interval of the first few years after separation or divorce, the continuation of which is dependent on the remarriage status of the former affine.

Summary

This paper has attempted to describe the current functioning of extended families and how that functioning is altered at the family level by the adaptation required in separation and divorce. A case study of a modern large and functional extended Jewish family has been presented in order to explore whether and how family membership changes after divorce. In this family which traditionally has tended toward open membership definition, the divorced/separated affines were included by 52% of respondents, although not as highly included as intermarrieds, a contrasting group. The reciprocally negotiated nature of the relationship after separation/divorce was stressed by many, as well as the elective nature of future relations based on ties of affinity. The results of this study also tend to confirm Spicer and Hampe's (1975) conclusions that being female and/or the presence of children becomes a functional equivalent of the marital bond. The specific findings here may have been influenced by the fact that divorced or separated affines were all female. Finally, this study may reflect a picture of the time interval just after separation and divorce, which may be essentially altered by the further passage of time and/or remarriage status of former affines.

REFERENCES

Bowen, M. *Family Therapy in Clinical Practice*. New York: Jason Aronson, 1978.

Leitcher, H.J. and Mitchell, W.E. "Jewish Extended Familism" in R.F. Winch and L.W. Goodman (Eds.) *Selected Studies in Marriage and the Family*. New York: Holt, Rinehart, and Winston, 1968.

Park, R. Jr. and Glick, P.C. "Prospective Changes in Marriage and the Family," *Journal of Marriage and the Family*, 1967, *29* (2) 249-256.

Parson, T. "The Kinship System of the Contemporary United States." *American Anthropologist*, 1943, *45*: 22-38.

Spicer, J. and Hampe, G. "Kinship Interaction After Divorce." *Journal of Marriage and the Family*. 1975, Feb. Vol. *37* (1): 113-119.

Sussman, M.B. and Burchinal, L. "Kin Family Network: Unheralded Structure in Current Conceptualization of Family Functioning." *Marriage and Family Living*, 1962, *24*: 231-240.

Uzoka, A.F. "The Myth of the Nuclear Family: Historical Background and Clinical Implications." *American Psychologist*, Vol. *34*, No. 11, Nov. 1979, 1095-1106.

Woodruff, R.A., Gize, S.B. and Clayton, P.J. "Divorce Among Psychiatric Outpatients." *British Journal of Psychiatry*, 1972, Sept. Vol. *121*, 289-292.

DIVORCE AND THE EXTENDED FAMILY: A CONSIDERATION OF SERVICES

Emily M. Brown

ABSTRACT. The impact of divorce on the extended family is extensive. Relatives, especially parents, experience feelings of disappointment, failure, and helplessness. They frequently provide extensive practical and economic support to the divorcing spouse who is related, often at a sacrifice. Except in regard to access to grandchildren, extended family members seldom request help from clinicians. If the needs of extended family members are to be met, clinicians will need to expand their definition of the divorcing family, and take an active role in reaching out to members of the extended family.

Divorce came of age in the 70's as a fact of life. Both the general public and professionals began to inquire into the phenomenon of divorce, and the emphasis shifted from preventing divorce to lessening the trauma of divorce. The divorcing family became the object of legal reforms, the subject of research, the recipient of specialized services, a favorite of the media, and a source of concern about the death of the family. The immediate family—the divorcing couple and their children—have been the focus of this attention. The 80's, with their increasing interest in family, provide a good opportunity to address the issues of divorce and the extended family.

Goode stated in 1956 that ''Neither the participants nor their close friends and relatives have been taught to react in a culturally approved

Emily M. Brown, MSW, is Director of the Divorce and Marital Stress Clinic in Arlington, Va.

fashion with respect to divorce.'' He later expressed the hope that his book might be useful to the kin of divorce ''who may give better advice, or may help more sympathetically, because they understand better what is taking place.'' (1965, p. vii)

A quarter of a century later, a great deal of attention is being given to divorce. Some of this is ''pop'' in nature, and some is genuinely helpful to those wanting to understand the process of divorce. Yet, it's seldom that the relationship between the divorcing couple and the extended family is even commented upon.

It's likely that this is due in part to our societal tendency to think in terms of family as the nuclear family, rather than the extended family. Another factor may be the norm we hold for kin relationships which Weiss describes as ''close but not too close''; loving, but neither confiding nor intruding; maintaining a separateness except in times of major change or need.

While it is generally accepted that the divorce experience is difficult at best for divorcing adults and their children, little has been said indicating that this is also true for the kin of the divorcing couple. The issues confronting the extended family are similar to those faced by the divorcing spouses. Both have to deal with emotional, social, and kinship issues, and it's common for both to be involved legally and economically as well. Thought the issues are similar,the experience of the extended family member is likely to be quite different than that of the divorcing spouse.

This article will describe some of the issues raised for the extended family by divorce, and will explore potential interventions. Most of the data is based on clinical observation with some additional information from selected interviews. The focus will be primarily on the period of time between the separation and the point a year or so later when new patterns become relatively stable. An operating assumption is that divorce generally has the greatest impact (particularly negative impact) on parents of the divorcing spouses, and a lessening impact as one moves outward in the family system to siblings, aunts, uncles, grandparents, cousins, and in-laws. The focus of this article will be limited to ''blood'' relatives, principally the parents.

Literature Review

Most of the literature on divorce and the extended family concentrates on the amount and kinds of support offered to the divorcing spouses and the changes in interaction within the larger family system. The findings tell us something about the impact of divorce on kin.

A study by Chiriboga indicates that although twenty-three percent of the divorcing men and almost a third of divorcing women seek advice and/or assistance (emotional support) from parents and relatives, only a very few found the parents or relatives to be the most helpful. In view of the very mixed feelings of extended family members to divorce, it is understandable that they may not be particularly emotionally supportive. Weiss (1975) noted that "Kin often insist on what they believe to be proper, irrespective of the wishes of the separated person."

Parents, however, provide a great deal of economic and practical support. Colletta, in a study of working class women found that single-parent mothers received assistance with child care mainly from their families of origin. This was true for over four-fifths of the low income mothers, and for two-thirds of the moderate income mothers. Financial help was given to 17% of the moderate income mothers and to 29% of the low income mothers by their parents. Other observers tend to agree that parents provide significant economic aid to divorcing daughters and sons; (Ross and Sawhill, 1975, Weiss, 1975). The effect of providing this help is not described but we might expect that it would be a sacrifice for most parents, that it may create an economical and physical strain for them, and probably some resentment.

It is likely that this situation is intensified when divorced offspring move in with parents. This is often a matter of economic necessity, and occurs more often in low-income families (Colletta). Although the literature does not report on the impact on the parents, it does indicate that living in the parents' household in an uncomfortable situation for the divorced daughter or son. Among female single parents, who moved in with their families after divorce, 86% were very displeased and worried about the tension it caused. (Colletta). Weiss reports that when this arrangement lasts more than a few weeks, it results in conflict. He also finds that daughters are more likely to be urged to return home than are sons; that daughters are viewed as "having tried adulthood and failed"; and that returning home is less of a problem for men because they don't become absorbed in the parents' household. He speculates that taking a divorced son or daughter in may be to compensate for guilt regarding the failed marriage, to have another chance to do better as a parent, or to turn back the clock by having the grandchildren in the house.

Spicer and Hampe, in examining kinship interaction after divorce, found that being female and/or having custody of children was associated with increasing or maintaining a high level of interaction with blood relatives, and with maintaining contact, although at a lower level, with in-laws. Former in-laws "are contacted when social variables define them as 'family'.'' Interaction with one's own relatives tended to stay the same, or for some, to increase.

Anspach, in a similar study, found that the ex-husband's kin were generally unlikely to have contact with the divorced wife, and could not be relied on for help unless the ex-husband intervened. The woman's own kin were most likely to be seen and provide help. Children's contact with the father's kin was dependent on the children's contact with the father. Over half the children who had contact with their fathers had as much contact with paternal grandparents as with maternal grandparents. However, in 69% of the households, paternal grandparents were seen less often than maternal grandparents.

Though it's clear that parents provide substantial support to their divorced sons and daughters, it is not known whether the amount or type of support has changed in recent years. Considering the large number of women who have returned to work after their children are grown, it is probable that parents these days provide more financial help and less in the way of help with household services such as child care.

Schlesinger suggests that the decline of the extended family may ''represent a greater loss for the one-parent family than it does for the two-parent family in that the former may be more likely to need the kinds of help and support which might be available from relatives in the home.'' (p. 3)

Underlying Emotional Issues

Underneath the immediate and apparent strains of a divorce in the family, lies a more basic issue. The questioning of family values, roles, and behavior patterns for both the divorcing person and his/her family. The choice of a spouse, and the roles and behavior patterns with the marriage are inextricably tied to the patterns learned in the family of origin. Moreover, parents often believe that if they've been good parents, their children will do better in life than they themselves have done (for their part, most children fully expect to improve on their parents). Parents devote significant levels of emotional and physical resources to making it possible for the kids to have a good life. As traditionally defined, the good life includes getting married, having kids, and ''living happily ever after.'' This belief, that marriage is central to the good life for their children, seems to be held whether the parents are happily married, have stuck out a bad marriage, or are divorced, and seems also to hold true within different cultural and socio-economic groups.

This belief is accentuated by our modern mythology, which gives gold stars for sticking it out, for not being a quitter, for making the best of a bad situation (reports of the "me generation" notwithstanding). These values contribute to our proclivity to view divorce as a matter of individual guilt or innocence. Thus, when a son or daughter divorces, many parents not only feel that their interest in the future is jeopardized, but that they have failed as parents. They may question their own life choices, struggle to avoid such uncomfortable issues, or experience resentment that a son or daughter can make a different choice. There is even shame at what others will say. There are concerns about family loyalties, and fear as to whether relationships with grandchildren and in-laws will be lost. There is anxiety about what roles to take with the son or daughter and with the in-laws, and apprehension about future demands on emotional and economic resources.

Siblings may feel virtuous in response to the separation of a brother or sister, or may feel threatened. Though the first divorce in a family is likely to evoke the strongest negative reaction, it is the subsequent ones which are likely to be interpreted by family members, especially siblings, as a predictor of their own marital failure. Even those who philosophically believe that divorce is better than a bad marriage find a divorce in the family upsetting.

Action and Reaction

Divorce pushes and pulls at the patterns of relationship within the extended family, and particularly at the ties between the divorcing spouses and their parents. Divorcing couples are well aware that relatives will react strongly to the news of an impending split. And they do: Such an announcement triggers immediate responses from kin, ranging from anger to bewilderment to solicitous concern, accompanied by everything from offers of material help to directives to lie in the bed one has made.

There are two typical patterns by which family members receive the news of an impending divorce. In the first, or support-building pattern, the husband or wife shares with a parent (or other relative) the fact that there is a problem in the marriage, and attempts (directly or indirectly) to line up that person's support. Variations of this pattern range from a straightforward message that says "We're having marriage problems, and I know you'll be upset if we can't work it out but I want your support," to "John is a dirty, rotten, no-good louse. I've done everything I can to be a good wife, and if we split up it's all his fault—I want you to take my side in getting even with him."

The second pattern features an announcement, usually at the last possible moment, typically just before or right at the time of separation. If parents live in another geographic area, it is very common for the announcement to them to be delayed until a month or more past the separation—when the son or daughter has gotten beyond the first few weeks of upheaval and trauma. When parents are elderly or in ill health, it is not uncommon for separated couples to hide the fact of the separation indefinitely, even to visiting parents together. Although a close sibling may have been in on the marital problems and the decision to divorce, and close friends probably were in on it too, parents are often among the last to know. Once they are informed they may get the job of giving other relatives the news. Often a chain reaction ensues, with parents informing others in a manner designed to elicit the least negative response. Those with closer family ties appear more likely to use a variation of the first pattern, while those whose families maintain more emotional distance tend to utilize the "announcement" pattern.

Upon the separation or its announcement, extended family members are faced with two major issues: How to deal with their own feelings and attitudes about the split, and how to respond. The initial reaction of relatives, especially parents, tends toward shock, disbelief, and sometimes non-acceptance. Out of their own shock and discomfort, family members often put the burden of proof on the divorced person.* Comments such as "Have you thought about your husband?" imply that the wife is being impulsive and put her on the defensive. If she tries to use the culturally accepted myth of blame to justify herself, her relatives are likely to find the situation unpleasant and may back off, blaming her for being non-objective, bitter, or selfish. A divorced woman in her 30's observed, wistfully, that when her relatives asked what happened, they "really only wanted one-liners" for answers.

It is a complex situation with relatives wanting explanations that will relieve their own anxieties and let them off the hook. Some insist, at the same time, that they don't want to get involved or take sides. Or, they may demand proof that the marriage was unbearable. A brother reports being surprised by his sister's separation. "I'd always regarded her as

---

*At a societal level, we often act like critical parents in response to divorce. We demand that the divorced justify themselves. This is most graphically illustrated in our legal system, which until recently required 'proof' of spousal fault and personal innocence as the only basis for divorce, and in some states still does.

the All-American wife and mother.'' Yet he also felt that her description of the situation was non-objective, ''it couldn't be all that bad.'' A divorced woman, watching her younger sister's marriage disintegrate, feels anquished at her own helplessness. ''It's like watching myself 10 years ago, and there's nothing I would have heard. Saying something to her would only make it worse.''

Weiss notes that ''We have no socially endorsed interpretation of separation to guide our response. Is it tragedy, failure, irresponsibility, the correction of a mistake, or just another change required by self-development? We know what it means if a spouse dies. But in response to separation, parents and siblings are likely to be uncertain.'' (p. 131)

It is obvious that parents care deeply about their divorcing children. However, they're in a position of relative helplessness to affect the turn of events. A father describes his reaction to his son's decision to divorce: ''It was quite a shock when it first came out, yet we were understanding of the circumstances. We realized he had tried for quite a period of time to do something about it, counseling and so on, and she wasn't receptive. It reached a point where he was concerned about his own health.''

A mother who had suspected something was wrong felt ''heartbreak for her rather than for myself'' on being told that her daughter was divorcing her husband because he was gay. ''The worst part was that she was hurting so much and there was so little I could do to help.'' The pain was mixed with relief that ''I've had an out for my daughter—it wasn't her fault, it's all because he's gay.'' She feels it would have been easier if she could have shared the reason for the split, but had gone along with her daughter's request to conceal the circumstances.

A mother who was raised to believe that when someone didn't want to live with a spouse, he or she shouldn't, reacted to her daughter's divorce: ''It was too bad for both of them. I did the proper thing—condoled with both of them, and wondered what had happened.''

The reaction to the split is also colored by the nature of the relationship with the spouse-in-law. When it's been a close one a divorce means loss, at least of some aspects of that relationship. For others as for a mother who had always found it hard to converse with her son-in-law, ''It was a relief not to have him as a responsibility.''

Reactions of parents and relatives tend to be typical of the family's style of interacting. Sadness, concern for both spouses, and offers of support come most often from families which normally function well and have strong emotional ties.

In those families where guilt and blame are important issues, ex-

tended familes often take sides and jump into the fray with a venge-
ance—usually on the side of the blood relative, but occasionally on the
side of the in-law. Other families react by avoiding discussion, involvement, and to some extent, contact with the divorced relative. Often
unresolved family issues are intensified. For example, in a family with a
domineering father and an acquiescent mother, the daughter's divorce
became a new issue in the ongoing power struggle. The father disowned
the daughter, forbade the mother to help the daughter, and effectively
became more dependent on the mother while cutting off any potential
benefits accruing from a relationship with their only child.

Most parents react with a mixture of feelings and behavior, as illustrated by the following case: Ann and her cousin, Lucy, grew up
together in Ohio and are close friends. As adults, each moved to Philadelphia. After five years of marriage and one child, Lucy was considering leaving her husband. She had never been able to talk freely to her
parents, and Ann suspects that Lucy's parents would not have been open
to hearing about Lucy's marital difficulties. As in earlier days, Ann was
Lucy's confidant, listening to Lucy's concern about the marriage, helping her clarify the issues, and sharing her perceptions of the situation, all
the while making sure that she didn't make the decision for Lucy. Ann
feels that Lucy needed her to talk to. "She needed to know that whatever
move she made, I would be there. I felt she definitely needed to get out of
the situation." Nevertheless, Ann described the experience as "one I
wouldn't want to go through again. I was apprehensive. I felt I had to be
careful so I wasn't responsible for her decision. I didn't want her to come
back later and say, 'Ann, it's all your fault—it would have worked out if
you hadn't told me to get out of the situation'." Lucy did decide to leave
her husband, and she and her 3-year old child moved in with Ann for a
month. Close to the end of the month she told her parents that she was
coming home to Ohio. For financial reasons she lived with her parents for
approximately one year. Her parents did little talking about the separation with Lucy, but what talking they did was directed toward getting her
to reconcile with her husband. They felt Lucy hadn't tried hard enough.
Lucy's mother tried to get information from Ann's mother (her sister-in-
law) so she'd know how to intervene more effectively. A year after the
separation, Lucy's parents became aware that Lucy's husband was having problems, and they urged her to go back to him at that time. Lucy
didn't want to return to her husband but felt confused by her parents'
pressure. Again, she confided in Ann, who responded that it would be
"an absolutely foolish move" and threatened to come to Ohio and

physically stop her. Lucy did not go to see her husband, nor did she reconcile. She has, however, stayed in touch with her husband's aunts and uncles. Her parents gradually gave up talking about the separation and the subsequent divorce, although Ann believes that they've never fully reconciled themselves to it. Looking back, Ann says, "I probably wouldn't have supported Lucy so much if I hadn't been so close to the situation and known what was happening." A postscript: Lucy's brother's wife is talking to Lucy about whether to separate. Ann advised Lucy to be careful, that listening to her sister-in-law could put her in an awkward position since Lucy's feelings were "bound to be with her brother." Ann summarizes the family's values: "Parents want kids to have a nice family, a nice home, and be on their own—to make it." She feels her parents would say "You're on your own now, you can come to me, but . . . you've got your own family."

In this family the major emotional support was provided by the cousin. Because Lucy had shared her situation with Ann over a period of time, Ann was not shocked about the eventual outcome, nor did she feel helpless. The critical factor, however, was the friendship, not the blood relationship. Despite their lack of approval, the parents came through with substantial economic and practical support by letting their daughter return home. The role of go-between adopted by the mother was not welcomed by the daughter—was a point of friction, and eventually was given up as unsuccessful.

Parents often find it possible to offer economic and practical support to a divorced daughter or son, even when they're unable to be emotionally supportive. Being able to offer some sort of aid may help parents cope with their feelings of helplessness about the divorce itself. It seems probable that those parents who are not able to cope with their helpless feelings are those most likely to distance themselves from their divorced sons and daughters. This appears to be true for siblings also and, to a lesser degree, for other relatives.

Providing practical help, is a mixed experience for parents. When a divorcing son or daughter returns to live with the parents it can be a particularly trying situation. A divorced father whose love relationship had just ended was glad to have his divorcing daughter and her child return home. "I needed something. It was a bad time for me. I thought she was going to stay two or three months but she ended up staying a year and a half. Most of that time I wished she was gone. After the first six months, I really began to feel deprived—of privacy, and having duties I didn't want. And then the little devil (granddaughter) became destructive. She began to tear up everything." Of his daughter he said that "she enjoys her privacy as much as I do mine," and believes that this motivated her to move out as soon as she was financially able to. He feels much better about doing the same types of things for her now than he did when she was there.

Women in particular are often unprepared financially to support themselves or their children. The mother of a woman who came home with two children states "our main objective for her was to get her on her feet—to get her so she'd be able to cope." As is common in this kind of situation the parents provided baby-sitting services and advice on child-rearing as well as food and shelter. This daughter also moved out as soon as she was financially able to do so, using a combination of some financial help from her parents.

The threat of losing contact with grandchildren comes up in some families, usually when the son or daughter is the non-custodial parent. This issue, more than any other, frightens grandparents. This may be because grandparents have little, if any, role in the outcome. For example, if the divorced son or daughter loses contact with the children, if the children live in another state, or if the non-custodial parent has visitation problems, grandparents are likely to feel frustrated and helpless. When there are no such barriers, or sometimes in spite of them, grandparents are willing to work on maintaining a relationship with grandchildren. In one instance, a grandfather whose son lives in another state, picks up his granddaughters regularly from his former daughter-in-law and has done so for six years. Although his wife never liked the daughter-in-law and does not see her at all, he maintained his friendship with her and never has a problem seeing his grandchildren even though the former daughter-in-law has remarried.

Summary of Issues

The issues confronting the extended family when a member divorces are many. The primary issues are emotional. Parents in particular experience feelings of disappointment, failure, and helplessness. They're often concerned about access to grandchildren. Siblings may jockey for a better position in the family, but may also feel threatened and helpless. Aunts, uncles, and cousins may be disapproving, or may be in the position of confidant—offering emotional support but feeling cautious about it. In addition, the extensive practical support offered by parents and relatives at times causes feelings of resentment or of being drained.

Interventions

Divorcing clients often call upon counselors and therapists as they struggle with the issues surfaced by a marital split, and with the reactions (real or anticipated) of parents and relatives. Despite evidence that extended family members, especially parents, are also upset by the divorce and are struggling with their own attitudes and feelings, few initiate a request for help.

Feelings triggered by the divorce (guilt, fear, ambivalence about their own marriage) may be regarded as unique or are suppressed. They may believe that the family should be able to handle its own problems. Parents are often ashamed, feeling that in some way their parenting has been faulty. The more traumatic feelings of their son or daughter may overshadow their discomfort. Despite evidence that extended family members, especially parents, are also upset by the divorce and are struggling with their own attitudes and feelings, few initiate a request for help. Some families are able to draw on internal skills and resources and don't need outside help. Others struggle less successfully by themselves for a variety of reasons, or they may not realize that help is available.

The one issue that does bring the extended family for help is that of access to grandchildren. The help requested includes legal information, counseling or mediation for the son or daughter and spouse-in-law, and, on occasion, counseling for the grandparent(s). Any other contact between extended family members and clinicians usually comes about when a divorced spouse invites relatives, usually parents, to be involved in the treatment process (generally as the suggestion of the therapist), or when relatives inquire about services and take an active role in referring the divorced spouse(s). Seldom, however, are the needs of the extended family members attended to.

Clinicians need to develop services which will help the extended family deal with divorce. Actually, many of the services now provided to divorcing spouses can easily be adapted to meet the needs of the extended family. A major need is for information: Information about the divorce process, about typical issues and reactions, about available resources, and on grandparenting and a variety of other topics. Seminars are a simple and effective way of providing such information. Seminars also provide some emotional support, and create an awareness that the issues are shared with others.

Clinicians working with divorcing individuals or couples are in an ideal position to help the extended family. Although quite often clinicians don't consider bringing relatives into the process or assume that relatives are not available, those who do reach out to the extended family generally find them to be quite willing to come in. The divorcing spouses may be more resistant to this approach than are the relatives.

Framo treats divorce "as a system problem that involves not only the immediate family but also the extended family and the rest of the couple's social network." He frequently brings in the couple's parents and siblings, and helps them examine how unresolved family problems are being acted out in the present. He believes, however, that "most therapists are not comfortable with the concerted unpleasantness of seeing several distraught family members together."

While not all families may be willing to participate in family therapy per se, many families may be able to benefit from several sessions with the therapist devoted to resolving specific issues. Even when the focus is on practical issues such as living arrangements, the clinician can be helpful by making interventions designed to reduce parents' feelings of failure. Suggestions for appropriate actions on the part of parents and relatives can serve to reduce feelings of helplessness. These might be suggestions for ways to share the pain of the divorce or ideas about practical support that might be welcomed. The therapist spotting power plays can surface the issues of loyalty and trust as important areas for further work.

When family therapy is not a possibility due to geographic distance, parents can be encouraged to talk to a knowledgeable clinician in their own community. In this situation, it is helpful if the clinician can make a referral.

Whether or not relatives are brought into the treatment process, clinicians can take an active role in educating divorcing clients. For example, therapists can help the client prepare to talk about divorce related issues with parents through techniques such as anticipatory exercises, rehearsal, and role play. Divorcing clients also need to become aware that they must take an active role with relatives. Clients might be encouraged, for instance, to tell relatives how they would like them to respond since, most often, relatives are uncertain as to how to respond. Clients can also be encouraged to share feelings such as disappointment about the end of the marriage in an adult way, rather than by retreating to the role of child.

Since parents and relatives are reluctant to initiate a request for help, it is not enough for clinicians just to be willing to offer services to the extended family. Clinicians need to take an active role. They need first of all, to identify the significant relatives of their clients and to reach out to them, either through the clients or directly. Then they need to function as a catalyst within the larger family system for the purpose of helping the family members resolve the emotional and practical issues surfaced by the divorce.

Clinicians also need to increase the visibility of services for the extended family, in ways that facilitate acceptance. For example, portraying extended family members as adjuncts to the therapeutic process or as members of a problem-solving team, is more conducive to involvement than is portraying them as the "identified patient." It is also important that descriptions of seminars emphasize the positive concern of the extended family rather than sore spots such as feelings of guilt or failure. Sensitive issues can be dealt with after a level of rapport has been established.

In talking about services for the extended family of divorcing spouses, we're really talking about expanding our definition of the client, rather than developing totally new techniques.

Much has been made of divorce as an opportunity for individual growth. The same holds true for the extended family: divorce provides an opportunity for the resolution of family issues. If not used, family issues may be exacerbated. Thus, it is important for clinicians to expand their conceptualization of divorcing families to include parents and other significant relatives.

BIBLIOGRAPHY

Anspach, Donald F. "Kinship and Divorce." *Journal of Marriage and Family*, vol. 38, No. 2. 1976. pp. 323-330.

Bohannan, Paul. *Divorce and After*. Garden City, New York: Doubleday. 1970.

Chiriboga, David A.; Anne Coho; Judith A. Stein; John Roberts. "Divorce, Stress and Social Supports: A Study in Helpseeking Behavior." *Journal of Divorce*, vol. 3, No. 2. 1979. p. 121-135.

Colletta, Nancy Donohue. "Support Systems After Divorce: Incidence and Impact." *Journal of Marriage and Family*, vol. 41, No. 4. 1979. p. 837-846.

Framo, James L. "The Friendly Divorce". *Psychology Today*, vol. 11, No. 9. February 1978. p. 77-79.

Goode, William J. *Women In Divorce*. New York: The Free Press. 1965.

Ross, Heather L.; Isabel V. Sawhill. *Time of Transition*. Washington, D.C.: The Urban Institute. 1975.

Schlesinger, Benjamin. *The One-Parent Family: Perspectives and Annotated Bibliography*. Third edition. Toronto, Canada: University of Toronto Press. 1975.

Spicer, Jerry W.; Gary D. Hampe. "Kinship Interaction After Divorce." *Journal of Marriage and Family*. vol. 37, No. 1. 1975. pp. 113-119.

Weiss, Robert S. 1975. *Marital Separation*. New York: Basic Books.